Understanding
Prostate Disease

This publication contains the opinions and ideas of its authors. It is intended to provide helpful and informative material on the subject matter covered. It is sold with the understanding that the authors and publisher are not engaged in rendering medical or other professional services in the book. If the reader requires personal medical or health assistance or advice, a competent professional should be consulted.

The authors and publisher specifically disclaim any responsibility for any liability, loss, or risk, personal or otherwise, which is incurred as a consequence, directly or indirectly, of the use and application of any of the contents of this book.

PEOPLE'S MEDICAL SOCIETY

Understanding Prostate Disease

Charles B. Inlander
Janet Worsley Norwood

Macmillan • USA

People's Medical Society is a nonprofit consumer health organization dedicated to the principles of better, more responsive and less expensive medical care. Organized in 1983, the People's Medical Society puts previously unavailable medical information into the hands of consumers so that they can make informed decisions about their own health care.

Membership in People's Medical Society is $20 a year and includes a subscription to the *People's Medical Society Newsletter*. For information, write to People's Medical Society, 462 Walnut Street, Allentown, PA 18102, or call 610-770-1670.

This and other People's Medical Society publications are available for quantity purchase at discount. Contact the People's Medical Society for details.

Many of the designations used by manufacturers and sellers to distinguish their products are claimed as trademarks. Where those designations appear in this book and People's Medical Society was aware of a trademark claim, the designations have been printed in initial capital letters (e.g., Cardura).

Macmillan General Reference USA
A Pearson Education Macmillan Company
1633 Broadway
New York, NY 10019-6785

Macmillan Publishing books may be purchased for business or sales promotional use. For information please write: Special Markets Department, Macmillan Publishing USA, 1633 Broadway, New York, NY 10019.

Copyright © 1999 by People's Medical Society

Library of Congress Cataloging-in-Publication Data

Inlander, Charles B.
   Understanding prostate disease / by Charles B. Inlander and Janet Worsley Norwood.
     p. cm.
   Includes bibliographical references and index.
   ISBN 0-02-862436-X (alk. paper)
   1. Prostate—Diseases—Popular works. I. Norwood, Janet Worsley. II. Title.
   RC899.I54   1999
   616.6'5—dc21   98-50713
                                                                         CIP

10 9 8 7 6 5 4 3 2 1

Printed in the United States of America

Contents

Introduction .... *ix*

Chapter 1 A Primer on the Prostate 1
    Anatomy of the Prostate 2
    Functions of the Prostate 4
    What Can Go Wrong 6
    Symptoms of Prostate Disease 7
    Finding the Right Practitioner 8
    Diagnosing Prostate Disease 12

Chapter 2 Dealing with Prostatitis 19
    What Is Prostatitis? 20
    Symptoms of Prostatitis 26
    Diagnosing Prostatitis 28
    Treating Prostatitis 29

Chapter 3 All About Benign Prostatic Hyperplasia 37
    What Is BPH? 38
    Incidence of BPH 39

    Causes of BPH 40
    Risk Factors for BPH 43
    Symptoms of BPH 45
    The Progression of BPH 46
    Diagnosing and Evaluating BPH 52

Chapter 4 Treatment for Benign Prostatic Hyperplasia 59
    Watchful Waiting 60
    Getting a Second Opinion 64
    Surgical Options 67
    Nonsurgical Options 88
    Medications 95
    Self-Care for BPH 104

Chapter 5 Understanding Prostate Cancer 109
    What Is Prostate Cancer? 110
    Incidence of Prostate Cancer 113
    Causes of Prostate Cancer 115
    Risk Factors for Prostate Cancer 116
    Preventing and Slowing Prostate Cancer 121
    Symptoms of Prostate Cancer 126
    Diagnosing Prostate Cancer 127
    Determining Cancer's Spread 142

Chapter 6 Treatment of Prostate Cancer 153
    Surgery: Radical Prostatectomy 157
    Cryosurgery 172
    Radiation Therapy 173
    Hormonal Therapy 179
    Drug Therapy 184
    Other Therapies 185
    Watchful Waiting 189
    Choosing Your Treatment According to Stage 194

  Follow-Up 200
  Recurrence 201
  The Emotional Effects of Cancer Treatment 203

Informational and Mutual-Aid Groups *211*
Glossary *213*
Suggested Reading *226*
Index *229*

Introduction

I'm frank to admit it, but like most men, I used to be paranoid about my prostate gland. It's hard to believe that such a small, almost minute part of the body could cause such anxiety. And it's especially surprising when you consider that about 20 years ago most men thought the word "prostate" meant to lie in a prone position (confusing it, of course, with the word "prostrate").

But there is no doubt about it. Today, every man age 40 and over worries that something will go wrong with his prostate gland. And why shouldn't we be concerned? It seems that every day we hear that a Bob Dole or a Norman Schwarzkopf or a Michael Milkin has been diagnosed with prostate cancer. Newspapers are filled with stories about new genes linked to prostate disease, new drugs in the pipeline that might shrink tumors, and new medical treatments that will replace last year's new treatments. There's hardly a family in the country that has not discovered prostate disease somewhere in the family tree.

Introduction

And on top of all that, the prostate gland has become an industry. Since the advent of the prostate-specific antigen (PSA) test, the number of prostate cancer cases has soared. It's not that the condition is invading the population at a faster rate than before, it's simply that now we can detect it sooner. That has made prostate disease a medical bonanza. Ten years ago, the radical prostatectomy (the surgical removal of the prostate gland) wasn't even one of the top 100 most often performed surgical procedures. Today, it is one of the top five. Most of these operations are performed on men over age 70, yet there are no studies suggesting there's much benefit to performing the operation on men that old.

There are urologists who concentrate solely on prostate problems. Most pharmaceutical companies are falling all over each other trying to find new drugs to treat prostate maladies. Shelves at health food stores are lined with herbal and other nontraditional remedies that tout themselves as prostate treatments.

While the prostate gland hasn't been the subject of a sitcom (yet!), it has certainly been the subject of hundreds of television news stories and specials. And each time a story appears, the media acts as if we've just had an invasion from Mars. The anchorperson becomes dour, footage of a worried elderly man resting in a recliner appears, and a vision of a white-coated doctor inevitably appears to tell us that there still may be hope.

So, of course, it's easy to be paranoid.

INTRODUCTION

But I'm also smart enough to know that most of our health fears are of the unknown. It's the lack of information that makes us worry most. The more I know about my prostate gland, what can go wrong with it, and what my options are, the less I have to worry. And after helping to write this book, my level of anxiety about prostate problems is down to zero. That's not to say that something might not go wrong with my prostate. In fact, the odds are that I'll develop any number of prostate problems. But I'm prepared for them because I have the facts I need to make an informed decision about what to do.

That's exactly why this book was written. The goal is to take the anxiety and fear out of prostate disease. We cover everything you need to know to better understand what goes wrong and what can be done about it.

And there is plenty of good news in this book. All forms of prostate disease—from gland enlargement to cancer—are treatable. Most of those treatments are successful for most men. There's also good news about what's on the horizon. Great advances are being made in prostate treatment.

The information you read in these pages comes from the most authoritative sources. We scoured the medical literature looking for the best studies on all aspects of prostate disease. This is not a book of opinion—it is a book of facts.

For more than 15 years, the nonprofit People's Medical Society has been the leading voice of the health care consumer.

INTRODUCTION

Our books and publications are the leaders in their field. And each one of our books is intended to empower you as a medical consumer. The more you know about your health, your conditions, and the medical delivery system, the better your chances of having a positive medical outcome.

Charles B. Inlander
President
People's Medical Society

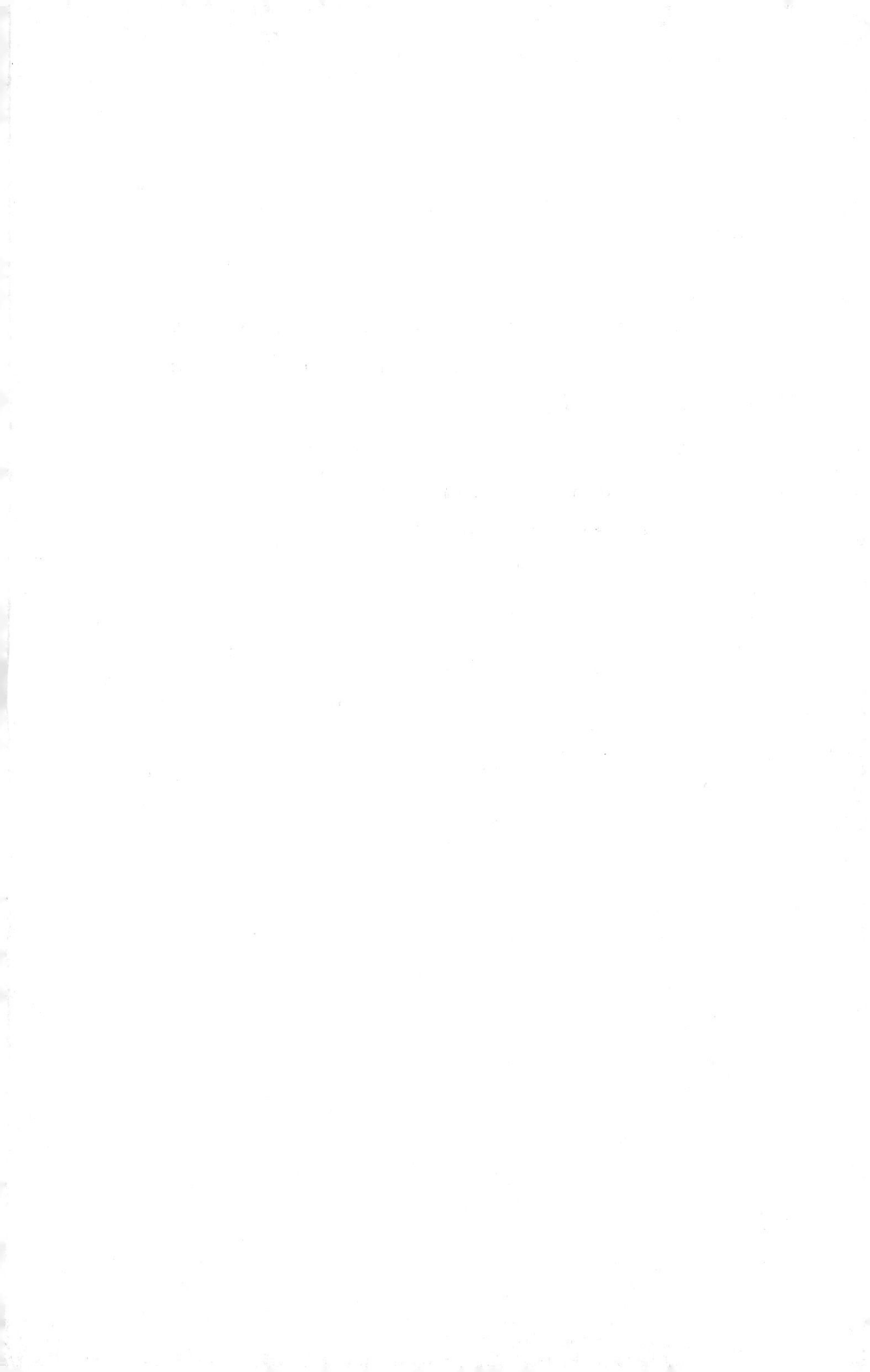

Terms printed in boldface can be found in the glossary, beginning on page 213. Only the first mention of the word in the text will be boldfaced.

We have tried to use male and female pronouns in an egalitarian manner throughout the book. Any imbalance in usage has been in the interest of readability.

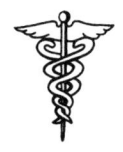

CHAPTER 1

A Primer on the Prostate

IF YOU'RE LIKE MOST PEOPLE, YOU'VE HEARD AT LEAST SOMETHING about prostate disease, and what you've heard may have been pretty frightening. After all, prostate disease—which includes **prostatitis, benign prostatic hyperplasia** (BPH, also known as enlarged prostate), and **prostate cancer**—is something to take seriously. More than half of all American men over age 50 are affected by enlarged prostates and the complications that come along with them. Approximately one in five American men will be diagnosed with prostate cancer in his lifetime, and some 39,200 die each year from the disease.

Without a doubt, prostate disease causes a lot of misery for a lot of men. But reading this book is probably one of the best ways to put your fears to rest. In these pages we present you with everything you need to know about prostate disease, from screening tests and symptoms to diagnosis and treatment, along with the latest scientific studies and evidence. Whether you're concerned about the possibility of prostate disease or are already dealing with it, we give you the information necessary for you to make the best decisions for your health.

Before we get into the details of prostate disease and what you can do to help keep your prostate as healthy as possible, let's take a look at exactly what the prostate gland is and how it functions.

Anatomy of the Prostate

The prostate gland is probably not what you think it is. Most people, if they've heard of the prostate at all, think it's a male sex organ. It's not, although it's in that vicinity and does play a role in the reproductive process. The **prostate** is actually a **gland,** a collection of specialized cells that secretes materials. It is part of the male reproductive system and is located in front of the **rectum** and at the base of the **bladder.** The prostate surrounds a part of the **urethra,** the tube that carries urine from the bladder out through the penis. The portion of the urethra that the prostate surrounds is called the **prostatic urethra.**

While we're on the subject of anatomy, here's a little more: The prostatic urethra ends at the external **urethral sphincter,** the muscle you voluntarily contract when you're urinating and want to stop the flow suddenly. There's another sphincter at the opening of the bladder, which operates involuntarily. Both function as valve mechanisms that provide urinary control in men.

In an adult male the prostate is about the size and shape of a large walnut and weighs about 20 grams, or a little less than an ounce. If you looked at the prostate under a microscope, you'd see a mass of muscle, glands, and connective tissue. The outer surface of the prostate is covered by thick muscle, often called the prostatic capsule because it encapsulates, or encases, the gland.

While there isn't any actual demarcation within the prostate itself, doctors often speak of the gland as being made up of "lobes" or "zones." The central zone surrounds the urethra. A larger, peripheral zone envelops the central zone. A transitional zone lies within the central zone, adjacent to the urethral sphincter. The transitional zone is small but medically important because it's within that area that problems may occur. When they examine the prostate for disease, doctors refer to these lobes or zones.

We'll talk about these structures and their functions in more detail as they come up, so don't worry if all of this anatomy and terminology seems a little confusing. The idea right now is just to become familiar with the terms—we'll fill in the blanks later.

Functions of the Prostate

Of course, now that you have some idea of where and what the prostate is, you need to know about how the prostate works. Again, the prostate is not a sex organ. As we said, it's a gland. But it's a pretty sexy gland, and its main role in life is sexual reproduction.

Let's start at the beginning. Around the same time that a boy's **testicles** develop the ability to produce sperm, the prostate gland becomes mature enough to produce the seminal fluid that will support the sperm. There are lots of small glands within the prostate, and they're producing and storing secretions more or less continuously. In fact, the prostate makes about 30 percent of the milky semen in which **spermatozoa,** the male reproductive cells, travel outside the body during orgasm and ejaculation.

At the risk of giving you another lesson in the birds and the bees, here's precisely what happens. Again, we go into more detail than you need right now because some of the anatomical parts we name here are going to play roles later in this book.

As every schoolboy knows, the testes manufacture sperm. The sperm are stored in a structure called the **epididymis,** located within the **scrotum.** During orgasm the sperm are pushed from their storage space into the prostatic urethra through two tubelike structures called the **vas deferens.** The sperm swim in fluid from the **seminal vesicles,** which are two saclike structures directly behind the base of the bladder. At the same time, the muscles of the prostate contract, pouring fluid into the prostatic urethra.

This broth of fluids is then propelled out, or ejaculated, by the spasmodic contractions of the muscles that surround the urethra. During sexual intercourse with a woman, the semen carries the sperm into the woman's vagina and uterus and up into the fallopian tubes in order to fertilize an egg.

In addition to supporting sperm as part of the semen, the prostatic fluid supplies some nourishment to the fragile sperm. It's also thought that this fluid helps make the vaginal canal less acidic. In these ways, the prostatic fluid works to increase the likelihood of conception.

The prostate gland does not play a role in sexual performance. It's a common misconception (if you'll excuse the pun) that men who develop prostatic problems can't have erections. The specter of **impotence** seems to loom over every uninformed discussion of the prostate.

The good news is that the vast majority of men who are treated for prostatic disease are able to perform as well sexually as they did before. The bad news is that in a minority of men, sexual performance is permanently impaired. As for fertility, obviously if there's no semen, there's no easy way of getting sperm to an egg. But there are other ways, and we address all these important issues later in more detail.

What Can Go Wrong

What goes on when there's a problem with the prostate? Three different types of disease affect the prostate gland. Two are **benign** conditions—that is, they're not cancerous. It's easy to confuse these three conditions, at least initially, because they produce many of the same symptoms.

Prostatitis is an inflammation of the prostate, often caused by a bacterial infection. While it is true that bacteria cause some types of prostatitis, no microbe has been held accountable for other types. Whatever its cause, prostatitis can occur in men of any age and generally responds to medication or other treatment.

Benign prostatic hyperplasia (BPH) is a noncancerous enlargement of the prostate. It's the most common type of prostatic disease: More than half of men over 50 have enlarged prostates.

The third disease is prostate cancer, which we mentioned earlier. It is a potentially serious disease because it's a malignant condition. That means that, over time, the cancer cells multiply without control, forming too much tissue and invading and destroying healthy cells nearby.

While prostate cancer can occur in men of all ages, 80 percent occurs in men who are 65 or older. Approximately one in five American men will be diagnosed with prostate cancer in his lifetime, and some 39,200 die each year from this disease, as we have mentioned earlier.

In this book we explore each of these diseases in detail. In Chapter 2 we talk about prostatitis. In Chapters 3 and 4 we discuss benign prostatic hyperplasia and its treatments. Chapters 4 and 5 are devoted to prostate cancer.

Symptoms of Prostate Disease

You can be alerted to prostate problems in a variety of ways—or not at all—depending on your individual situation. Distinguishing among prostate conditions is often difficult because many of the symptoms are similar.

The most common symptom is a urinary problem. You may find that you need to urinate more often, especially at night. You may have trouble starting the urine flow. Once it's started, you may have trouble stopping it; urine may trickle out, stop, and start again. Depending on the particular disease, you may have pain or burning when you urinate, chills, fever, and pain in the lower back, pelvis, or upper thighs. You may also have watery or brownish discharges from your penis that are different from the secretions your prostate normally produces. Sometimes you may have **hematuria,** or blood in the urine.

It is possible, however, to develop a prostatic disease and have no symptoms for a while. That's particularly true with cancer of the prostate, which grows slowly and in its early stages typically doesn't produce any symptoms that signal its presence. Because prostate cancer tends to be "silent," routine tests are available to help catch cases early.

Finding the Right Practitioner

If you suspect that you have a prostate disease or want to be tested, seek a medical opinion from your primary care physician. You also have the option of seeing a **urologist**—a specialist in men's urinary and reproductive system health (although if you're involved in a managed care plan, you may need to check with your primary care, "gatekeeper" doctor first).

If you're facing prostate disease, whether it be prostatitis or prostate cancer, you need to find a physician you trust to provide your care. In some cases, mild prostate disease may be handled by a primary care physician—that's the doctor who handles your everyday ailments, such as a cold or the flu. In many cases, however, prostate conditions benefit most from the expertise of a specialist.

A specialist is a doctor who concentrates on a specific body system, age group, or disorder. In the world of medicine, prostate conditions are treated—along with other reproductive and urinary disorders in men—by a specialist known as a urologist. To become a urologist, an M.D. (doctor of medicine) or D.O. (doctor of osteopathy) must undergo two to three years of supervised specialty training (called a residency). Often a specialist also takes one or more years of additional training (called a fellowship) in a specific area of the specialty, called a subspecialty.

How can you tell if a doctor is a trained specialist? A doctor who has taken extra training in a field often chooses to become board certified. In addition to the extra training, the doctor must pass a rigorous examination administered by a specialty board, a national board of professionals in that specialty field. A doctor who passes the board examination is given the status of diplomate. Most board-certified doctors become members of their medical specialty societies, and any doctor who meets the full requirements for membership is called a "fellow" of the society and may use the designation.

In its most basic sense, board certification indicates that a physician has completed a course of study in accordance with the established educational standards. Board certification has been called a minimum standard of excellence and nothing more. Paper certification does not produce professional excellence. On the other hand, board certification is a good sign that the person is up-to-date on the procedures, theories, and success-failure rates in the specialty. There are, however, some inferior doctors who somehow manage to become board certified and some excellent doctors without board certification.

The training requirements are similar for M.D.'s and D.O.'s, although certification is usually by different boards. M.D.'s are certified by one or more of the 24 member boards of the

American Board of Medical Specialties (ABMS); D.O.'s are certified by the department of certification of the American Osteopathic Association (AOA). In the case of urology, however, both osteopathic and allopathic physicians are certified by the American Board of Urology, an allopathic board, as there is no osteopathic board designated for urology.

The training programs for ABMS-recognized specialties are offered only at accredited medical schools with approved programs. There are also self-designated medical specialty boards, which are not recognized by the ABMS or the AOA and may not have the same standards and training requirements as the national boards.

You can find the names of many board-certified specialists in *The Official ABMS Directory of Board-Certified Medical Specialists* and the *American Medical Directory: Physicians in the United States,* both usually found in local libraries. The ABMS directory will also tell you where the doctor did his residency training and how long he has been practicing.

If you wish to call to verify the credentials of a specialist, you can contact the American Board of Medical Specialties at 800-776-CERT. For more information on osteopathic certification, contact the American Osteopathic Association, Department of Certification, 142 East Ontario Street, Chicago, IL 60611; 800-621-1773 or 312-280-5845.

The Search for the Perfect Practitioner

If you don't have a urologist and hope to get one, begin your search by getting a few good recommendations from family members, friends, and neighbors. Don't overlook your primary care provider, either. Other sources to consider are:

- Physician referral services operated by the local medical society (usually county based) and local hospitals. However, such services will refer only those practitioners who are members and will not comment on the ability of providers other than perhaps to mention their board certifications.

- Your company personnel office. Companies sometimes use certain practitioners for employment physicals and disability claims.

- Health insurance companies, which can sometimes be helpful when you require a specialist for a second opinion.

- Listings in the telephone directory. Practitioners' names are usually arranged according to practice or specialty, but remember that a doctor can practice in any specialty area he or she chooses, whether or not he or she has had any advanced training. Look for board certification.

continues

> - Nurses or other medical professionals
> - Senior centers. Some have lists of practitioners either affiliated with or recommended by the center.

THE ROLE OF THE PRIMARY CARE PHYSICIAN

An April 1997 survey in the *Journal of General Internal Medicine* reported that more primary care practitioners than ever were taking care of patients with benign prostatic hyperplasia. However, according to the survey, primary care practitioners were less likely to use the diagnostic methods recommended by the Agency for Health Care Policy and Research (AHCPR), an authoritative federal organization that evaluates standards and guidelines, than urologists were—either because they disagreed with the AHCPR's guidelines or because they weren't familiar with them.

Diagnosing Prostate Disease

Whether you decide to visit your primary care practitioner or a urologist, several tests may be done to detect prostate disease, regardless of your symptoms. While some of these tests are helpful only in pinpointing a specific prostate disease, others can be used to help diagnose more than one condition. These tests will be mentioned throughout this book, so to help you along, here's a brief rundown of the most common diagnostic methods.

Questions to Ask

Once you've decided what type of practitioner you would like to visit and you've found a few in your area, the next step is a face-to-face meeting. Call the office for an appointment and mention that you may be a new patient, then ask to arrange a get-acquainted visit, a 15-minute meeting at which you can ask questions and find out a little more about the practitioner. Be aware that some practitioners charge for these appointments.

During the visit, evaluate the office and staff. Ask a receptionist about the procedures for making appointments, telephoning the practitioner, getting prescription refills, and obtaining copies of medical records.

Because the meeting with the practitioner is short, have your questions ready. You will want to know the practitioner's medical degree, board certification, and hospital affiliations. Ask about fees and payment plans.

This is also an opportunity to discover the philosophy of the practitioner: What is the attitude toward alternative therapies? Is the patient viewed as a full partner in health care? Also notice the demeanor of the practitioner: Are your questions heard and answered in a forthright manner? You will also want to consider:

- Is the practice solo or group?
- If group, are the practitioners in the same specialty?

continues

- If group, are the practitioners in different specialties?
- Does this practitioner publish or make available a list of fees and current charges?
- Does the office appear neat and clean? Are there current magazines?
- Is your insurance coverage accepted? Will the office file all insurance claims?
- Does the staff maintain a professional, friendly attitude?
- Was your appointment kept on time?

URINALYSIS

One of the most basic and common tests available is **urinalysis**. An analysis of your urine can show whether any bacteria or white cells are present, indicating infection.

The urine test may be a somewhat elaborate, three-cup process that allows the doctor to analyze the first urine you void, your "midstream" urine, and a third sample that contains prostatic fluid.

If you report trouble urinating, the doctor may use a machine to measure your urine flow rate. She may also insert a **catheter**—a long rubber tube—into the bladder through the urethra to measure **urinary retention**.

DIGITAL (MANUAL) RECTAL EXAM

A **digital (manual) rectal exam** is a simple, relatively painless—but often uncomfortable—exam that takes about a minute and can be done by either your family doctor or a urologist. While you bend at the waist and lean over an examining table or chair, the doctor inserts a lubricated, gloved finger up your rectum to the point where he can feel your prostate.

A rectal exam may reveal a great deal. A normal prostate feels smooth and elastic. The presence of lumps or other areas of abnormal texture, or a prostate that's rock hard, may well point to cancer. If the prostate is enlarged, it could indicate the onset of benign prostatic hyperplasia (BPH). We discuss BPH in detail in Chapter 3.

It is recommended that you have routine rectal exams. It is through this exam that most cases of prostate enlargement are first identified and some cases of prostate cancer are first diagnosed. The exam is such a standard and important part of men's health care that it's sometimes known as the "male Pap smear," after the widely used screening test for cervical cancer in women.

There's considerable disagreement over the age at which a man should have his first rectal exam and how frequently such exams should take place after that. The American Cancer Society (ACS) recommends a rectal exam each year for all men over age 50—or younger if they're in any high-risk groups.

Some health authorities, not including the ACS, think that men who are age 70 or older and have no symptoms can give up routine rectal exams, because the prostatic cancer the doctor would be looking for tends to progress so slowly that the men are likely to die first of other causes.

Some groups feel that men should forgo rectal exams altogether because they may not be helpful in detecting prostate cancer and may lead to unnecessary testing. In fact, the latest *Guide to Clinical Preventive Services,* issued by the U.S. Preventive Services Task Force in 1995, comes out against all routine rectal exams or other tests for prostate cancer. We talk about all of these tests and their advantages and disadvantages in Chapter 5.

CYSTOSCOPY

Another urological test is called a **cystoscopy**. It's a procedure that involves passing a cystoscope—a slender, hollow tube with a light and a lens on one end and a viewing lens on the other—through the opening in the penis, into the urethra and then into the bladder. The procedure can be done with a local anesthetic and, if you're especially nervous, a sedative as well.

Cystoscopy is an exceptionally valuable procedure because it helps doctors diagnose most of the diseases that affect the prostate. By looking through various lenses, doctors can see the interior of the prostatic urethra and diagnose inflammation.

If a prostate is enlarged, cystoscopy can indicate the degree of obstruction in the prostatic urethra, the size and weight of the obstructing prostatic tissue, and any urinary retention (or how much urine is retained in the bladder because it can't get through the urethra). The cystoscope is also used in men with prostatic cancer to locate sources of prostatic bleeding and to assess how much the tumor is impinging on the urethra.

A cystoscopy sounds pretty awful, but most men who've undergone the exam say the anticipation is worse than the reality. The newest cystoscopes are more flexible than the original models, making them less uncomfortable. However, you should be aware that cystoscopy, like any procedure of this type, carries a relatively small risk of infection. Rarely, injury to the urethra—which may lead to the formation of scar tissue that interferes with urination—occurs during the procedure.

In many cases, other tests serve the purpose just as well. Some urologists perform cystoscopy only under special circumstances, such as to evaluate blood in a person's urine.

OTHER TESTS

Blood tests and x-rays may also be done. Quite a few blood tests evaluate how well the kidneys are functioning and look for prostate cancer. One that you'll read a lot about in this book is called the prostate-specific antigen (PSA) test, which we have more to say about in Chapter 5.

> ## At a Glance: Commonly Used Diagnostic Tests for Prostate Disease
>
> **Digital (manual) rectal exam.** A procedure in which a doctor inserts a gloved, lubricated finger into the rectum and, through the wall of the rectum, checks the prostate for hard or lumpy areas.
>
> **Cystoscopy.** A procedure in which a cystoscope—a slender, hollow tube with a lens at each end—is passed into the penile urethra and bladder, allowing visual examination of the urinary tract.
>
> **Urinalysis.** The physical, chemical, and microscopic analysis of urine for abnormalities.
>
> **Prostate-specific antigen (PSA) test.** A test for prostate-specific antigen, a substance that is produced exclusively by prostate cells and whose level increases in the presence of prostatic cancer and rises significantly with metastasis, or spread, of the cancer.

Imaging and **biopsy** are two other diagnostic tools that can help to determine the presence or extent of prostate cancer or can provide information about the urinary tract prior to surgery.

Next, we will get into more detail about the different types of prostate disease, starting with prostatitis.

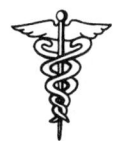

Chapter 2

Dealing with Prostatitis

OF ALL OF THE MOST COMMON CONDITIONS THAT CAN AFFECT THE prostate, prostatitis is generally the most transient and the least serious—if treated promptly. Strictly speaking, prostatitis is an inflammation of the prostate. Bacteria or some other microorganism can cause the condition, or it can result from factors other than bacteria. As we say in Chapter 1, prostatitis is a benign condition, meaning that it is not cancerous. Most cases of prostatitis can be successfully eradicated with medications or other treatments.

In this chapter we give you a rundown on the types of prostatitis that might cause you problems, followed by information on symptoms, diagnosis, and treatment.

What Is Prostatitis?

There are two kinds of prostatitis: nonbacterial, or noninfectious; and bacterial, or infectious. We'll cut out some of the medical verbiage and refer to the two categories from here on as **nonbacterial prostatitis** and **bacterial prostatitis**. But first we should note that *prostatitis* is often used as a catchall term for a handful of different urinary tract infections and conditions. Because of the way the urethra, bladder, and prostate are connected, conditions affecting one or another often have similar or overlapping symptoms.

NONBACTERIAL PROSTATITIS

Nonbacterial prostatitis is the most common kind of prostatitis and, as its name suggests, isn't a disease (a specific illness or disorder) or an infection (which is caused by a virus or bacteria) but is, rather, a health condition—a problem that affects the state of the body. Doctors generally divide nonbacterial prostatitis into two categories: **Congestive prostatitis** (sometimes called **prostatostasis**—literally, "condition of the prostate") is the more common; the other is **prostatodynia** (which means "painful prostate").

Congestive Prostatitis

Congestive prostatitis occurs when too much prostatic fluid, the milky liquid that goes into semen, accumulates within the prostate gland rather than being ejaculated out of the body. It's said that the prostate is "congested" or "engorged."

Some practitioners believe that chronic, unrelenting stress is responsible for most cases of prostatic disease in which the prostate becomes congested, particularly when there's no sign of bacteria or a virus. And some scientists are still searching for a mystery microorganism.

But in the absence of other evidence, other eminent urologists have concluded that sex—too much or too little—is to blame for congestive prostatitis. That's the hunch of Stephen N. Rous, M.D., author of *The Prostate Book,* and the late Monroe E. Greenberger, M.D., author of *What Every Man Should Know About His Prostate.*

Remember that old husbands' tale (we'll call it that because we're sure it wasn't an old wives' tale!) that a man could become ill if he didn't have enough sex? Some caddish fellows used it to persuade reluctant virgins to go to bed with them. Well, in these experts' view, there may be some truth to the story.

What's the physiological basis for this presumption? Every day a healthy prostate secretes between one-tenth and two-fifths teaspoon of prostatic fluid. When you're sexually aroused, however, you produce between 4 and 10 times that amount. Normally, you release it through ejaculation. But if you don't ejaculate, the fluid builds up and the prostate becomes congested.

Men who never ejaculate aren't necessarily doomed to congestive prostatitis. Nonbacterial prostatitis has been called the disease of popes and priests, but it's probably caused more by an abrupt change in sexual habits than by celibacy. Suppose you're used to ejaculating on a fairly regular basis of, say, three times weekly. Then, for whatever reason—maybe you had a falling out with your sexual partner or one of you is ill or traveling—the rate drops to once a week or less. Your prostate gland has become "programmed" to secrete merrily at the three-times-a-week rate, but now the fluid has nowhere to go. So the gland swells up.

The prostate can also be irritated by too much sex. Suppose you've been celibate for a long period, then have an extremely active weekend. Your prostate, which has become used to a low rate of secretion, is suddenly required to produce fluid for several ejaculations. This isn't a case of a congested prostate, just an extremely irritated one.

There are theories of other causes of prostatitis. Greenberger has suggested that the condition can also be caused by **coitus interruptus**—the practice of withdrawing during intercourse before orgasm occurs—which may diminish the volume of ejaculation, and by chronic vibration, which seems to give the prostate the illusion that intercourse is imminent and leads it to secrete fluid. Bus drivers and motorcycle police are among the people whose jobs predispose them to congestive prostatitis.

Prostatodynia

Prostatodynia is the term used to describe a condition in which pain seems to be originating in the prostate, but it is much more likely to be coming from the muscles of the floor of the pelvis, from an inflammation in one or more of the pelvic bones, or from a disease in the rectum. In this condition, the prostate itself is probably normal.

The cause of prostatodynia is not clear, although some physicians think it's stress related. Sometimes examinations show that the bladder neck and urethral sphincter—one of the muscles that control urination—are hypertonic, or tense. Ira Sharlip, M.D., a urologist and assistant clinical professor at the University of California Medical Center in San Francisco, has said that, in the absence of bacteria, "most prostatitis is actually urinary sphincter hypertonicity."

BACTERIAL PROSTATITIS

Bacterial prostatitis is easy enough to define: a prostatic disease caused by a bacterial infection in the prostate. And like the nonbacterial variety, bacterial prostatitis takes two forms: acute and chronic. Both are fairly uncommon.

Acute bacterial prostatitis is a rare and serious illness, not to be confused with the garden-variety prostatic conditions we've just described. It results from a sudden infusion of bacteria into the prostate gland, either by direct extension from an infection in the urethra or, very occasionally, by a blood-borne spread of bacteria from an infection elsewhere in the body.

Chronic bacterial prostatitis is, as the name suggests, a recurring infection in the prostate. It's probably the result of residual infection when acute bacterial prostatitis hasn't been knocked out of the system.

Bacteria that are in the colon, called **colon bacilli,** are the cause of most common prostatic infections—and remember, bacterial prostatitis is relatively uncommon. The bacteria get into the prostate directly from the rectum or through the bloodstream. You can acquire the bacteria by swimming in unclean pools or beaches or by drinking dirty water. It's also possible, although unlikely, to pick it up from a bacterial infection elsewhere in the body, such as a sinus infection, tonsillitis, an abscessed tooth, or an ear infection. In such cases, the bacteria are borne by the blood.

You can also develop bacterial prostatitis if you already have an enlarged prostate, or the condition known as BPH, which is so common in older men. When the prostate reaches a certain size, the obstruction may make it impossible for you to empty your bladder completely. Bacteria can grow in the stagnant urine that remains. That may lead to a bladder infection, which occasionally spreads to the prostate. By the same token, you're at a higher risk for getting bacterial prostatitis if you've recently had a urinary catheter inserted to drain urine from your bladder.

Bacterial prostatitis cannot be sexually transmitted. Although bacterial prostatitis is an infection, it's not contagious. So you can't give it to your sexual partner. However, a number of infections transmitted during sexual intercourse, including **gonorrhea** and candida—the latter a common infection that you probably know as a yeast infection—can lead to bacterial prostatitis. Infection can also be transmitted through anal intercourse because it can send bacteria-laden feces into the bloodstream.

It might sound like it's pretty easy to get infected, but in reality it is not. The prostate is in a capsule that's not easily penetrated, so it's fairly well protected against infections. But when microorganisms do get in, they find the prostate is a good host. The **blood-prostate barrier,** which keeps certain substances from penetrating the prostate, also keeps out most antibiotics. So once the prostate is infected, it can be extremely difficult to eradicate bacteria—hence the chronic, recurring tendencies of the condition.

OTHER FORMS OF PROSTATITIS

Although the conditions we've just discussed are the only ones truly considered to be prostatitis, the term is often applied to other conditions with similar symptoms. The main one is **nonspecific urethritis (NSU),** a fairly common infection of the prostatic urethra. It's usually caused by **chlamydia,** the most frequently reported infectious disease in the United States. However, other bugs can work the same mischief.

Urethritis, if left untreated, may progress to a kidney infection, but fortunately it's generally caught long before then. For our purposes here, the most important thing about urethritis is that it can lead to acute bacterial prostatitis.

Symptoms of Prostatitis

Although there are some variations, both nonbacterial and bacterial prostatitis share many of the same symptoms. With both conditions you might find that your penis seems to be "glued" shut when you wake up in the morning. When you open it, you'll probably notice a drop or two of clear liquid. At the end of the day, you may find a brownish or yellowish stain, about the size of a dime or a quarter, in your underpants.

You may also get a feeling of discomfort or itching deep inside your penis. And you may feel some discomfort when you urinate. How bad is the pain? Well, if you've had much to do with the medical profession, you've probably concluded that discomfort is a popular euphemism for pain. But if you've ever urinated with a kidney stone, you know the difference.

Because of symptoms such as itching and dripping, it is easy to confuse prostatitis with a sexually transmitted disease—a problem that's complicated by the fact that gonorrhea can lead to prostatitis. However, the early signs of the two conditions are different. Gonorrhea affects what's called the anterior portion of the urethra, the part that's within the penis rather than the part that's enclosed by the prostate. So if you have gonorrhea, the itching and discomfort will be toward the end of your penis.

Other symptoms may occur depending on the condition. If it's nonbacterial prostatitis, the prostate may be swollen or engorged. Temporarily, that creates the same problem you encounter with benign prostatic hyperplasia: It becomes difficult to urinate.

With prostatodynia, there's usually pain or discomfort in the **perineum** (the area between the scrotum and the **anus**), in the rectum, or in the area just above the pubic hair line.

With acute bacterial prostatitis, symptoms may become severe. In that case, you can run a fever of 102°F or higher. You may have malaise, the aches and pains usually associated with flu. And often you'll develop low abdominal or lower-back pain. The infection makes the prostate gland swell too, so it may be difficult or even impossible to urinate.

With the exception of acute bacterial prostatitis, prostatitis is not a serious condition. Having prostatitis doesn't increase your risk of getting any other prostatic disease, including cancer. Nor does it lead to impotence.

This does not mean, however, that you can skip a trip to the doctor. Because the symptoms of the various forms of prostatitis, except acute bacterial prostatitis, are so similar, it's important to undergo tests that pinpoint a diagnosis—the subject of the next section of this chapter. Once you figure out what you've got, we'll discuss how to treat both bacterial and nonbacterial prostatitis.

Diagnosing Prostatitis

When diagnosing prostatitis, the first thing a doctor will do is perform a rectal exam. If the prostate feels somewhat enlarged and spongy, you could have nonbacterial prostatitis. And if the sexual history you provide shows a recent erratic pattern, that's confirmation.

If you're showing signs of acute bacterial prostatitis, however, the doctor should perform the rectal exam gingerly or perhaps not at all. For one thing, the prostate will be extremely tender and painful. But more important, too much pressure on the prostate might propel the infection into the testicles, epididymis, or bloodstream, causing severe **systemic** infection.

In addition to the rectal exam, your physician will almost certainly do a urinalysis to check for signs of infection, such as white cells and bacteria. A culture is done of the urine sample to encourage microorganisms within the urine to grow so they can be identified. If your urine has a high bacteria count, you probably have acute bacterial prostatitis.

It is somewhat harder to diagnose chronic bacterial prostatitis. For this diagnosis your practitioner will need a slightly more elaborate test—actually a series of tests called a **segmented urine culture.** First, you'll urinate into a cup. Then you'll do a midstream urination. Next, the doctor will insert his gloved finger into your rectum and massage, or "strip," the prostate to force a few drops of prostatic fluid into the urinary tract. This isn't a painful procedure, but it is fairly uncomfortable. Finally, you'll urinate into a third cup. Because of the prostatic massage, the third urine sample will contain prostatic fluid.

The doctor will culture all three urine samples. If the urine sample containing prostatic fluid has a high bacteria count, a diagnosis of chronic bacterial prostatitis is reasonable. On the other hand, if the bacteria counts for the first and third urine samples are equally high, it's probably urethritis rather than prostatitis.

Rarely is a cystoscopy—the viewing procedure we discuss in Chapter 1—necessary in the diagnosis of prostatitis. A cystoscopy could show inflammation of the prostatic urethra, which would confirm a diagnosis of urethritis or possible bacterial prostatitis. But in the vast majority of cases, a careful urinalysis should suffice.

Treating Prostatitis

Nonbacterial and bacterial prostatitis are handled in different ways, and your options may vary according to the type and severity of your condition.

NONBACTERIAL PROSTATITIS TREATMENTS

In the case of nonbacterial prostatitis, antibiotics are useless because there are no bacteria to be eradicated. Unfortunately, there's almost a knee-jerk reaction that, when prostatitis is diagnosed, antibiotics are called for. In fact, a 1994 study from Massachusetts General Hospital in Boston found that—despite the researchers' estimate that only 5 percent of cases of prostatitis are bacterial—45 percent of men with prostatitis symptoms receive prescriptions for antibiotics.

At times physicians do prescribe antibiotics to cover all the bases in case a hidden infection has been overlooked. However, most people won't respond to antibiotics because there's actually no infection and no bacteria. They run the risk of being on antibiotics for months—at unnecessary cost and possibly at the expense of developing side effects and later antibiotic resistance—and yet still have the problem.

If not antibiotics, then what? For congestive prostatitis, both Greenberger and Rous say you should treat yourself to a sexual romp in bed. After all, if the condition is the result of a buildup of fluid, the remedy is to release the fluid, that is, to ejaculate.

If that's not an option, these urologists add, then take matters into your own hands, so to speak. Some men who are reluctant to masturbate may feel less guilt-ridden if they know they're doing so on doctor's orders.

If neither sex nor masturbation is possible, another option is prostate massage, which we described earlier as part of the test for prostatitis and which can be done in a doctor's office. Like ejaculation, it has the effect of releasing seminal fluid and relieving congestion.

To date, no drugs have proved useful for treating nonbacterial prostatitis. A 1996 study published in the *Journal of Urology* reported that the drug allopurinol (most commonly used to treat gout) eased symptoms of nonbacterial prostatitis. Although many physicians now prescribe allopurinol in hopes it will be effective, others have criticized the study as flawed and unreliable.

For prostatodynia, a condition that's often thought to be stress related, treatments focus on relaxation. In some cases, doctors may recommend tranquilizers or psychotherapy. **Alpha-adrenergic blockers,** which you'll read more about later in the discussion of BPH, are also sometimes used for prostatodynia because they relax the smooth tissue in the prostate and bladder neck. The drug most often used is called prazosin (brand name Minipress, manufactured by Pfizer) because it is available in low doses and has fewer side effects than other options.

If the pelvic area appears inflamed, doctors may recommend over-the-counter anti-inflammatory medications such as ibuprofen or aspirin. Another popular treatment for prostatodynia is a hot sitz bath, which draws more blood to the area, increases local circulation, and relaxes the muscles. Biofeedback has also helped some people.

In addition to medical treatments, a number of self-help remedies may help relieve prostatitis. There's what doctors call anecdotal evidence—based on patients' reports rather than on clinical studies—that certain beverages, such as coffee, gin, whiskey, and red wine, and spicy foods irritate the prostate and can promote a flare-up of prostatitis. (It may not be coincidental that these same drinks and foods also irritate the bladder.) Some men also report that heavy lifting, vigorous exercise, and especially prolonged driving can worsen the symptoms.

You should not ignore the symptoms of prostatitis. With nonbacterial prostatitis, it's possible to grin and bear it. But apart from the fact that there's no point in suffering pain needlessly, there's some evidence that nonbacterial prostatitis can make a man more susceptible to bacterial prostatitis. And a study by Israeli researchers indicated that this condition, in some men, may damage the sperm and result in sterility.

BACTERIAL PROSTATITIS TREATMENTS

The treatment of bacterial prostatitis usually calls for antibiotics. Before you start a course of antibiotics, however, you first need to make sure you've got a bacterial infection. Chances are, you don't: As we said earlier, bacterial prostatitis is fairly uncommon. Only a handful of cases of prostatitis actually involve bacteria. Think twice if your physician writes you a prescription without doing a urinalysis. A complete **urine culture** is usually necessary to make a proper diagnosis.

For acute bacterial prostatitis, you typically take antibiotics for several weeks. Depending on how severe the symptoms are, you may also be put on **analgesics** to relieve pain and be ordered to rest in bed. You may even be hospitalized and put on intravenous antibiotics because of the danger that the infection might spread to the bloodstream. Or you may be hospitalized if your prostate is so swollen as a result of the infection that you're completely unable to urinate, or if you need intravenous fluids because you're running a high fever.

Expect there to be careful follow-up. The problem with this particular infection is that it's virtually impossible to be sure it's cured. So you may find it coming back, time and again, as chronic bacterial prostatitis, and each time it will be more difficult to cure.

Men who develop chronic bacterial prostatitis are usually treated with a combination of sulfa and trimethoprim (examples of brand names are Bactrim and Septra) or with other drugs, depending upon the bacteria's sensitivity to antibiotics. If the infection is particularly stubborn, a man may stay on antibiotics for three months or more. There are cases in which men have been on continuous antibiotic therapy for years. Researchers are also starting to look at the possibility of combining antibiotics with alpha-adrenergic blockers, which relax the smooth tissue in the prostate and bladder neck, for better results.

For particularly resistant cases of chronic bacterial prostatitis, researchers are investigating the injection of antibiotics directly into the prostate. One small 1996 study from Japan reported a complete cure of bacterial prostatitis for 56 percent of its 25 patients with one or two antibiotic injections, although the authors stressed further research is needed to prove the merits of the method. While the treatment can be somewhat uncomfortable, the benefits probably outweigh the discomfort of the injections or the risk of long-term antibiotic therapy. However, the therapy is still very experimental at this point.

In extreme cases, your doctor may advise either a partial or a complete **prostatectomy,** or surgical removal of the prostate. Surgery might be called for if you're developing urinary retention or kidney problems as a result of prostatitis. Or maybe, because you've had frequent prostate infections, you've acquired a tendency to develop stones in the gland. The stones then become contaminated, and that perpetuates the prostatitis. Clearly, surgery is the last resort. Surgical options are discussed in depth in Chapter 4.

Medical options aside, there are some self-help remedies that may help treat bacterial prostatitis. Some experts believe that zinc may act as a defense against prostate infection, for both prevention and therapy. Zinc is found in high concentration in seminal fluid and in the prostate itself. In fact, there's more zinc in the prostate than in any other place in the body.

Researchers have found that, in the laboratory, the amount of zinc normally present in prostatic fluid is effective against various types of bacteria. At the same time, they've noted that patients with chronic prostatitis have either little or no zinc in their prostatic secretions. Some experts believe that the drop in zinc concentration precedes any bacterial invasion, rather than bacteria causing a drop in zinc levels.

There's considerable debate over whether zinc is effective. Many researchers believe that the prostate does not pick up zinc from the bloodstream when it's taken in pill form (as a supplement would be taken). Having said that, we'll add that another school of thought believes zinc supplements to be worthwhile. Those researchers recommend zinc sulfate tablets in doses of 50 milligrams a day (zinc gluconate, which many people take to fight colds, is not effective). You can also eat zinc-rich foods such as oysters, nuts, pumpkin seeds, wheat germ and bran, milk, eggs, chicken, peas, lentils, and beef liver. (Of course, some of those foods are also high in fat and cholesterol and are to be avoided for that reason.)

Certain individuals need more zinc than others: people with diabetes, heavy drinkers, and, according to some doctors, people undergoing unusual stress. Before you step up your dosage of zinc, however, you should consult a physician—or, if alcohol is the issue, cut back your drinking.

And some doctors warn that, while small amounts of zinc may boost the body's immune system, extremely large amounts may make it more difficult for the body to defend itself against infection.

Another favored self-help remedy is cold-pressed linseed oil, a homeopathic treatment. Another treatment is a pollen preparation called cernitin. Both therapies are available at drug and health food stores. For more information about such remedies, consult homeopathy guides and your local health food store.

For the most part, however, prostatitis—as prostate conditions go—isn't often very serious. The other conditions—benign prostatic hyperplasia and prostate cancer—generally cause more concern. We'll talk about BPH next.

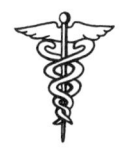

CHAPTER 3

All About Benign Prostatic Hyperplasia

BENIGN PROSTATIC HYPERPLASIA (BPH) MEANS DIFFERENT THINGS to different people. To health professionals, benign prostatic hyperplasia is a noncancerous enlargement of the prostate gland. (In medical lingo, the term *hyperplasia* refers to an increase in the number of normal cells in an organ or tissue, so that the organ or tissue grows in size.)

To men with BPH (as we'll call it from here on), the condition is more personal than any definition can convey. BPH may mean repeated nighttime trips to the bathroom, annoying drips and drabs of urine at inopportune times, or a nagging feeling that a visit to the men's room is necessary. If BPH progresses, it may partly or completely block urination. In its least common, most serious forms, BPH invites kidney damage and failure.

Unfortunately, there's no denying that BPH is a common condition, though most sufferers face only mild symptoms. It's been said that BPH accounts for urinary problems in about 10 million men in the United States over age 50. According to the National Center for Health Statistics, each year the condition is responsible for 1.7 million doctor's office visits and some 400,000 operations. The good news is that more can be done today than ever before to help slow the progression and treat the symptoms of BPH.

What Is BPH?

In BPH the prostate is actually growing. When a boy is born, his prostate is about the size of a pea. It grows very slowly until puberty, when there's a period of rapid growth that continues for several years, until the prostate reaches its normal adult size. It remains that size until about age 40 or 45. At that point the prostate begins to grow again and continues growing until death.

On average, it might grow as large as 33 grams, or 1.5 ounces. That's fairly small. Still, it's an increase of 50 percent over the prostate's normal size. (The largest reported prostate size in a man with BPH was 1,058 grams, but that's the stuff of medical case studies.)

BPH is not cancer. As the term itself says, the condition is benign, not malignant. If you looked at both normal prostate tissue and BPH tissue under a microscope, you'd see that BPH tissue generally has more glandular tissue and less muscle and connective tissue. But for all practical purposes, there's no difference between the two kinds of tissue.

Even so, prostate growth means trouble. As they say in real estate, it all comes down to location, location, location. Because of its placement in the body, an enlarged prostate can have a stranglehold on the urethra.

Think of the urethra as a straw that runs from the bladder to the end of the penis, draining urine from the body. BPH begins right up against the wall of the prostatic urethra (the part of the urethra that passes through the prostate). If growth is outward, away from the urethra, or even if the prostate becomes as large as a tennis ball, it's not a problem. But if the new growth is inward, the prostate presses in on the urethra, squeezing it and making urination increasingly difficult.

Incidence of BPH

BPH is very common, and becoming more so all the time as life expectancy rises. It's been called the disease of old men—one of the most famous prostate patients in recent years was President Ronald Reagan, who, at the age of 76, had surgery for BPH in 1987—but it afflicts plenty of not-so-old men too.

Statistically, the odds of a man developing BPH are quite high. However, in the flurry of numbers, it might sound as though any man who lives long enough to grow a few gray hairs is doomed. So it's useful to distinguish between an obstructive prostate and one that's merely enlarged. Autopsy studies show that more than half of all men who are age 50 or over and about three-quarters of men who are age 70 or over have BPH. By age 80, the incidence is even higher.

That doesn't mean that the men died from the condition—just that it was present when they died. It also doesn't mean that the enlargement was progressive or that they had any symptoms. Stephen N. Rous, M.D., estimates in *The Prostate Book* that between one-quarter and one-half "of those men who have anatomic changes of BPH will also have the symptoms which will send them to their physicians." That averages out to about one in six men over age 50 and about one in three over age 70. That's a minority, but it's still a big number.

Causes of BPH

Two groups of men are impervious to BPH, and their characteristics provide us with a lot of information about the causes of BPH and how it might be treated.

One group includes men who've been castrated—that is, they've had their testicles removed surgically or shrunk by taking female hormones such as **estrogen** and no longer produce

testosterone. These men's immunity to BPH led doctors years ago to the conclusion that enlargement of the prostate gland is somehow related to the production of testosterone.

About 100 years ago, in fact, men with obstructive BPH were sometimes castrated as a way of relieving their symptoms, and doctors boasted that their patients improved at rates of 80 to 87 percent. Once surgical remedies were introduced, castration was out.

The second group consists of men who have normal testosterone levels but in whom BPH just does not develop. Not only do these men have small prostates throughout their lives, but their prostates actually decrease slowly in volume as they age. Although in other ways the men are normal, they have less facial and less body hair than the average male, and they don't grow bald.

It's been found that these men have a genetically linked deficiency of an enzyme called **5-alpha-reductase.** That enzyme converts testosterone into a more active **androgen,** or male hormone, called **dihydrotestosterone (DHT).** Because they lack this enzyme, testosterone cannot be converted into DHT.

Because men who lack DHT don't suffer from BPH, many experts believe this hormone has much to do with the development of an enlarged prostate. The concentration of DHT in the normal prostate and in seminal vesicles is much higher than in other tissues. And DHT concentrations in BPH tissue that's removed during surgery are higher than those seen in normal prostate tissue. Moreover, in test-tube studies, DHT has been shown to stimulate hyperplasia in prostate cells.

Most animals lose their ability to produce DHT as they age. Men produce less testosterone as they age, but they continue to produce and accumulate high levels of DHT in the prostate.

The belief is that DHT is transported to the nuclei of the prostate cells, where it sets off a cascade of events that ultimately stimulate the production of proteins called **growth factors.** These factors act on prostate tissue to cause the enlargement known as BPH. Studies have shown that BPH tissue has more growth factors than normal prostatic tissue.

In addition to testosterone, it's believed that estrogen may also be a causative factor in BPH. Men's bodies normally make a certain amount of estrogen, which, along with testosterone, stimulates normal prostate tissue. As men age, they produce less testosterone and relatively more estrogen. Studies done with animals suggest that the higher amounts of estrogen in the prostates of older men may increase the activity of substances that make the cells grow.

No strong evidence exists that BPH runs in families. In other words, it's probably not hereditary in the traditional sense. However, some researchers think BPH may develop as a result of genetic programming—"instructions" given to cells early in life. In this theory, BPH occurs because cells in one section of the gland follow these instructions and "reawaken" later in life. These "reawakened" cells then deliver signals to other cells in the gland, instructing them to grow or making them more sensitive to hormones that influence growth.

Another theory on the cause of BPH involves the tissue of the prostate. Some scientists believe that, in addition to hormonal factors, the nervous system is sending messages to tighten up the prostate's muscle tone. And that means increased pressure on the urethra.

Here's how. As much as 60 percent of the prostatic tissue in people with BPH is **stroma**—that is, tissue that makes up the framework of the gland—and a substantial portion of stromal tissue is made up of muscle. Under an electron microscope, the stromal tissue appears to have larger cells than the prostatic tissue of men who don't have BPH.

Some scientists believe that receptors in the stromal tissue respond to signals from the nervous system and heighten prostatic muscle tone. One group of researchers has suggested that as much as 40 percent of the urethral closure pressure in men with BPH is due to stimulation of prostatic muscles.

Risk Factors for BPH

There is little that can be done to prevent BPH from developing. Apart from testosterone, researchers haven't identified any special risk factors in men who eventually develop BPH. They can't blame the usual suspects, such as smoking, caffeine, or obesity. Sexual habits and previous infections don't seem to make any difference. About the only practice that has been clearly implicated in the development of BPH is the use of anabolic steroids by athletes and others who are active in bodybuilding.

One study did find that the risk of BPH seemed to decrease among men who drank between two and four beers a day. Before you head out for a six-pack, however, you should be aware that there's no clear cause and effect. The study questioned men who'd already had surgery for BPH, so it's possible that they changed their drinking habits after their conditions developed. Or drinking may correspond to other factors such as diet.

Experts are not sure if diet has an impact on the risk of BPH, and there are no hard data to say it does. It's worth noting, however, that the incidence of BPH among Asian men has historically been very low and has risen significantly as the men have moved to the West or changed their traditional lifestyles. Since Asians tend to have a low-cholesterol, low-fat diet, American men who want to avoid BPH (not to mention heart disease and other health problems) might wish to follow their example.

Having BPH does not increase your risk of prostate cancer. It's true that the two often appear together, but that's only because both diseases are fairly common in older men. Men with enlarged prostates subsequently develop cancer at the same rate as men with normal-size glands do.

When men have surgery for BPH, a procedure we describe in the next chapter, the tissue removed is routinely checked for hidden cancer cells. In about one out of 10 cases, some cancer tissue is found. Often, however, it's limited to a few cells of a nonaggressive type of cancer, and no treatment is needed.

Symptoms of BPH

A number of symptoms are associated with BPH. Generally, they arise at different stages of the condition. But even if your prostate enlarges to the point where you need to seek surgical or other treatment, you won't necessarily have all the symptoms. And even if you have all the symptoms, you don't necessarily have BPH.

Now that you're forewarned, here's a list of what you can expect:

- More frequent urination, especially at night
- Some difficulty beginning urination
- A urine stream that's weak and thin
- Difficulty stopping urination abruptly, often followed by a persistent "dribbling"
- A feeling that you need to urinate urgently
- A feeling that your bladder hasn't completely emptied
- Urinary retention (inability to urinate)

Blood in the urine is another common symptom. In fact, BPH is one of the most common causes of hematuria in men over 40. You can develop hematuria when the urethral blood vessels and the bladder neck get stretched so much by the growing prostate tissue that they burst.

If a very small blood vessel ruptures, there may be only a microscopic trace of blood in the urine. But if it's a larger blood vessel, the urine will turn pink or red. It's rare but possible for a severe hemorrhage to take place. When that happens, you've got to take care of the condition immediately—seek emergency care.

The Progression of BPH

BPH is a progressive disease, meaning that it slowly grows worse. When BPH first begins, you probably won't realize that your prostate is growing. The condition develops so gradually that it's generally years before you realize there's a problem.

As the prostate grows, it begins to encroach on the urethra. Initially, the bladder compensates for the narrowed urethra by contracting more forcefully than before to push urine through. To do this, the bladder muscle—like any muscle that has to work overtime—thickens, particularly just inside the bladder neck and on the floor of the bladder.

As long as the bladder muscle can overcome the resistance put up by the growing prostate and narrowed urethra, the bladder can empty itself every time you go to the bathroom. In this stage, your bladder is said to be **compensated,** and you don't have any symptoms of BPH.

Symptoms set in during the months and years after the onset of BPH. As the bladder muscle builds and thickens, the floor of the bladder becomes more sensitive to the presence of urine. As a result, you feel the need to urinate more often. Most men notice this initially at night, when they're awakened by the need to go to the bathroom, so the symptom is called **nocturia.**

As a rule, your bladder can accommodate about 5 ounces of urine before you feel the need to void. When you're sleeping, you can generally tolerate even more than that without waking up. Furthermore, when you're asleep, the amount of urine your kidneys produce—generally about 2 ounces each hour when you're awake—falls off. That's why most people can sleep a full eight hours without going to the bathroom.

Once nocturia begins, however, considerably less than 5 ounces will sound nature's call. As the bladder grows more and more sensitive, you'll wake up once, twice, five times a night.

Of course, this sensitivity doesn't end when the sun rises. You'll probably feel the need to urinate more frequently during the day too. But that's a feeling people can ignore more easily when they're up and about. It's when you're sleeping, even when you're dreaming, that your brain pays prompt attention.

As BPH progresses, you'll probably start to notice the condition during the day as well. This usually occurs when your bladder can no longer push effectively past the obstructing prostate. Because the bladder muscle is straining against the resistance of the prostate, you'll start noticing that it takes several seconds to a couple of minutes for your urine flow to start. When the stream finally starts, it's "hesitant" and weak. This condition is called **hesitancy.**

You're particularly likely to run into this situation if you've waited a long time to urinate. Maybe you've been on a long car trip, or you've refused to budge from your seat during an especially riveting football game. Your bladder may become overstretched, and since it has gradually lost its tone, it contracts only weakly.

As BPH progresses and the muscles of the bladder continue to build, complications may occur. For example, bands of scar tissue, called **trabeculations,** eventually begin to form in the bladder wall. In more advanced cases of BPH, weaker areas of the bladder wall between the areas of trabeculation begin to bulge outward, creating little sacs or pouches called **cellules.**

Eventually the cellules balloon and form small pouches, called **diverticula,** that can trap urine and become a home for bacteria. If you've developed trabeculations and diverticula, you may still have urinary problems even after you've been treated for BPH.

Urinary problems may also persist if your bladder muscle has deteriorated to the point where it's permanently weakened. In that case, you can expect to continue to have a problem with urinary retention.

As the bladder muscle starts to weaken, an annoying phenomenon that doctors call **intermittency**—what most men refer to as dribbling—occurs. As the obstruction grows, your bladder eventually can't empty itself completely with a single muscle contraction. Your stream of urine stops before your bladder is empty. Seconds later the muscle contracts a second time, weakly, and the stream starts again.

Sometimes this occurs near the end of the stream. You think you're through urinating, so you zip up. Then a few drops to an ounce or more of urine may dribble onto your underwear.

As the condition progresses, the bladder becomes **decompensated.** It can't empty, even with a second contraction, so some residual urine is always present. (Under normal conditions, a bladder empties itself almost completely.)

Once the residual urine in the bladder reaches 3 or 4 ounces, you notice that it's only a short time after voiding that you feel the need to void again. You may be voiding every 30 minutes to two hours. You may also become unusually susceptible to bladder or kidney infections. The collecting urine is stagnant, so it's a perfect culture for growing bacteria. If this happens, you begin to feel burning pain when urinating. Often your urine acquires what some people call a barnyard smell. In addition, some men develop bladder stones. Sometimes they're extremely painful, and sometimes so insignificant they aren't bothersome at all.

As the residual urine builds up to a pint or more, there's no room left in the bladder for new urine coming down from the kidneys, and urine involuntarily leaks from the urethra, usually when you're asleep. This is an advanced stage of BPH.

Having all that urine in the bladder is uncomfortable and potentially dangerous, and complications can occur. If urine can't leave the bladder through the urethra, eventually **reflux** pressure backs the urine into the kidneys. That makes it impossible for the kidneys, which should be filtering and removing various waste products from the body, to do their job. This condition can result in kidney damage and, more rarely still, kidney failure. A condition called **uremic poisoning** can result, which, if left untreated, can lead to coma and death.

Uremic poisoning can be prevented by regularly monitoring kidney function. Doctors recommend that all men with BPH get a blood test as part of their yearly checkup, to determine how well their kidneys are functioning. The test reveals your levels of **creatinine** and **urea nitrogen,** two of the waste products that the kidneys are supposed to flush constantly out of your blood. If the creatinine level is abnormally high—which may occur if you've had a major problem with residual urine for a long time—that usually means the kidneys have already been damaged.

If the kidneys continue to function and if the condition isn't too severe, some men can live with urinary retention indefinitely. But other men eventually arrive at a painful state called **acute urinary retention.** That's when they're completely unable to urinate.

Acute urinary retention can be brought on suddenly in men with only moderate BPH who take over-the-counter cold remedies or allergy medicines. Cold and allergy medicines may contain antihistamines, which block nerve impulses. Other cold and allergy medications contain a decongestant drug known as a **sympathomimetic,** which may, as a side effect, tighten the bladder neck and make it difficult to urinate. (These medications don't usually have this effect on younger people.)

When there's a partial obstruction, urinary retention can also be brought on by alcohol, cold temperatures, or a long period of immobility, such as being confined to a bed or wheelchair or simply sitting for several hours.

Acute urinary retention is treated at a doctor's office or the emergency department of a hospital. The condition can be alleviated easily and quickly; a doctor inserts a catheter into the penis to drain the urine directly from the bladder. Relief is immediate. If you haven't urinated for 12 hours or more, as much as 4 quarts of urine may pour out.

In most cases, urinary retention occurs long after BPH has been diagnosed. There are times, however, when it might take a man by surprise. It's hard to believe, but very occasionally a man may not be aware he has an obstruction until it becomes completely impossible for him to urinate.

This condition—the combination of acute urinary retention and asymptomatic obstruction—is called **silent prostatism.** For several days before the crisis develops, as the man's kidneys fail, he may become extremely weak, sleepy, and irritable. Without warning, he may suddenly become comatose. Unless he has his bladder drained immediately, he can die.

One explanation for why you may have an obstruction and not know it is that BPH can develop so gradually that you can get used to the symptoms to the point where you can't remember when you didn't have them. Or maybe you're denying the problem because you don't want anybody tinkering with that part of your anatomy.

Diagnosing and Evaluating BPH

Not every urinary problem can be attributed to BPH. All the symptoms we've listed above, particularly residual urine, often occur in elderly women. Obviously, they can't blame the prostate for their conditions.

The symptoms that are characteristic of BPH can also be caused by urethral **stricture** or scarring, bladder problems, inflammation, infection, or other conditions, such as neurological disorders. Diabetes also can lead to frequent urination and can interfere with sexual performance. It's not unusual for a man to think he has prostate problems when he's really showing signs of diabetes. The same problems can also be caused by some of those medications we mentioned earlier, such as antihistamines or decongestants, that can interfere with bladder function.

The point we're trying to make here is that it is important to seek out a diagnosis if you have urinary problems. If there's a possibility that you have any of the conditions we just mentioned, particularly if you're under 55, you should have a series of diagnostic tests to determine bladder function. The prostate isn't always to blame, either. For example, according to several studies, about one-third of men who are told that their **incontinence** is due to prostate enlargement actually learn from **urodynamic studies** that there's an altogether different cause.

Doctors can pinpoint BPH and evaluate its progression in a number of ways. They start by taking a history that includes information about your sexual habits. They want to know, for example, whether you've ever had a sexually transmitted disease, which can result in symptoms similar to those seen in prostate disorders. They also want to know how often you urinate and whether there's been any change in the pattern.

Because it's hard to give more than a subjective account, you can help the diagnostic process by monitoring your urinary habits and symptoms before the visit. On a sheet of paper, write down four urinary symptoms (you can take any of the several symptoms we enumerated earlier). Each day put a check for each time the problem occurs. After one week you'll have a factual record to present to the doctor.

A physical exam also helps to diagnose BPH, though it is not as valuable as other diagnostic methods. In such an exam, the doctor may press down on your bladder to determine whether it's full of urine and distended. He's also likely to do a rectal exam, though that's of limited use in detecting BPH. The rectal exam indicates whether the prostate is enlarged but not whether it's causing urinary symptoms. You see, the part of the prostate that generally causes obstruction is the middle lobe, or central zone, and that's what tightens around the urethra. Unfortunately, that's the part that can never be felt during a rectal exam.

Another problem with the rectal exam is that the overall size of the prostate doesn't necessarily indicate the stage of BPH. As a rule, the size of the prostate doesn't reflect how severe the obstruction is. Some men with greatly enlarged prostates have little obstruction and few symptoms, while others whose glands are less enlarged have more blockage and greater problems.

To find out more, the doctor will probably do a urinalysis and urine culture to look for infection. The presence of red blood cells suggests problems in the urinary tract, such as stones or tumors, but it may also indicate BPH. White blood cells or pus may indicate infection or inflammation in the kidneys, the bladder, or the **ureters,** the tubes that carry urine between the two organs.

He may also conduct a urodynamic evaluation, which may consist of a urine flow test and a residual urine test. To measure urine flow, he'll use either a machine called a **uroflometer** or just a stopwatch and a measuring container; you'll contribute a full bladder. The doctor will measure what you think is your strongest flow, and compare it with the standard flow rate for your age group. Men over 60 should have a flow rate greater than 13 milliliters per second, for example, compared with 22 milliliters per second for men under 40. A slow flow rate may indicate BPH, but it may sometimes be due to weak bladder muscles, not to prostate problems. Other tests may be necessary.

One such test, for residual urine, is done with a **bladder catheterization.** After you've emptied your bladder (or think you have), the doctor inserts a catheter into the bladder for a few minutes to measure the amount of residual urine. In theory, the more residual urine, the greater the need for treatment of BPH. However, residual urine can also indicate a weak bladder muscle.

One other note regarding bladder catheterization: When most people hear the word *catheter,* they tend to think of the **Foley catheter.** However, the catheter used here is a simple "in-and-out" catheter, not a Foley catheter, which is designed to be left in the bladder for long periods of time and stays inside with the help of an inflatable bag that catches on the bladder neck. There are many different reasons for using Foley catheters, but in the case of BPH, they're normally inserted when the prostate is so large that a man can't urinate at all. As a rule, the Foley catheter remains only until the obstruction is resolved. But it may remain indefinitely if the patient refuses to be treated or his medical condition is so poor that he's considered a poor risk for surgery.

Blood tests may be performed as part of the diagnostic process as well. Although there aren't any blood tests for BPH, there are tests for related conditions. We've already mentioned the blood tests for kidney function. There are two other blood tests, for **prostatic acid phosphatase (PAP)** and for prostate-specific antigen (PSA) levels, that are routinely performed on men being examined for BPH. The primary purpose of both these tests is to detect prostate cancer. You can expect some blood tests during the exam and certainly before any surgery takes place. We describe the PSA test at greater length in Chapter 5. Let us just say here that the results of the PSA test must be handled with care. Men with enlarged prostates tend to have elevated PSA readings, which can also indicate the presence of prostate cancer. So if you have a high PSA level, you may be subjected to other tests—and a lot of worry—until it can be determined that the only problem is BPH.

X-rays may also be used at times. Some urologists take an **excretory urogram,** also known as an **intravenous pyelogram (IVP)** or **intravenous urogram (IVU),** which provides a lot of information about the entire urinary tract. It's performed by injecting (into a vein in the forearm) a dye that concentrates in the kidneys and appears white against the dark background of an x-ray.

The dye's passage through the system over the course of half an hour is recorded on a series of films. The test shows how well a patient empties his bladder, reveals any obstruction to the drainage of the kidneys, and even indicates the size of the prostate through a shadow it casts within the bladder. However, there's a major drawback to IVPs. People have had serious—and occasionally even fatal—allergic reactions to the dye. One explanation may be that iodine is the base of some of the injected material. It's almost impossible to predict who will have a bad reaction, so an alternative dye has been developed. Because it's extremely expensive, many urologists prefer to use other tests.

Other tests that might be done if you're being examined for BPH include **renal scans** and **ultrasound.** Renal scans, produced after injecting a very small amount of radioactive material, give a picture of the kidneys. So does ultrasound, a totally noninvasive procedure that is generally considered one of the safest tests. But while ultrasound can help estimate the size of the prostate, it doesn't help you or your doctor decide whether surgery or other treatment is actually needed. That's because prostate size isn't an indication of the extent of obstruction.

A cystoscope lets a doctor see the degree of obstruction in the prostatic urethra and estimate the size and weight of the obstructing prostatic tissue. This test helps determine how best to treat BPH if surgery is recommended. The doctor will also be able to measure any residual urine that may be present, since the urine will come out through the cystoscope after it has entered the bladder. The test also shows changes in the bladder, such as the trabeculations we spoke of earlier. But the test cannot determine whether you actually need treatment for BPH—that is, whether the obstruction is bothersome. That's up to you.

While none of the tests and examinations we've described is conclusive alone, as a group they can confirm a diagnosis of BPH. They can also help determine the extent of the enlargement and evaluate its effect on your urinary health. Once you have this information in mind, you can use it to sort out your treatment options—the subject of our next chapter.

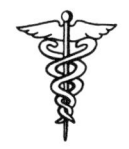

CHAPTER 4

Treatment for Benign Prostatic Hyperplasia

IF YOUR DOCTOR TELLS YOU THAT YOU HAVE BPH, THEN IT'S TIME to get down to practicalities. What should you do? Maybe nothing, maybe a whole lot. The first thing you should know is that an enlarged prostate alone is not reason enough to undergo treatment. It's generally agreed in the medical community that BPH requires treatment only if either of two conditions apply: The symptoms are severe enough to be bothersome (for example, you continually feel the urge to urinate and you're retaining large amounts of urine), or the function of the urinary tract is seriously affected.

If your condition is uncomfortable or dangerous, you've got an almost bewildering number of possibilities: surgical procedures, less invasive procedures such as balloon urethroplasty, and a fairly recent but important addition, medications. The field is changing rapidly, and so are your options. What you choose to do depends on your objectives, age, general health, symptoms, and, of course, your insurance coverage and economic condition.

Your choice also depends on your doctor's advice. Certainly you should get her opinion, as well as a second and maybe a third. You'll find there's a lot of honest confusion and disagreement among physicians about when and how to treat BPH. This is borne out by a study several years ago by John Wennberg, M.D., M.P.H., of the Dartmouth Medical School. It found that, from one community to another, the probability that an older man would undergo surgery for BPH varied by more than threefold.

This chapter, which describes treatments ranging from the nontreatment approach of watchful waiting to invasive surgical options, is designed to help you sort through the maze of alternatives available. With this book as a tool, you'll be able to choose the treatment that is best for you.

Watchful Waiting

Perhaps your symptoms are only moderate. You need to urinate a couple of times during the night, and your flow is weaker—and tests indicate that your bladder and kidneys aren't in any immediate danger. In that case, you may opt for what the medical profession calls "watchful waiting"—that is, you do nothing more than have regular checkups to make sure that the condition isn't worsening and that you're not developing complications from BPH.

No dictum says your condition will inevitably grow worse. In a 1992 issue of *American Health* magazine, Aaron Kirkemo, M.D., a urologist at Henry Ford Hospital in Detroit, noted that "a significant number of men with symptoms will not need surgery. Prostate symptoms fluctuate over time; some get worse, but some get better with no treatment at all."

One indication of how your condition may progress may be the severity of your initial symptoms. A January 1997 study of watchful waiting, reported in the *Journal of Urology,* found that 83 percent of men with mild symptoms who chose watchful waiting had the same mild symptoms four years down the road. Fifty-nine percent of men with moderate symptoms continued to have moderate symptoms. However, only 33 percent of men with initially severe symptoms stuck with watchful waiting, while 40 percent underwent surgery for prostate troubles.

In an effort to promote understanding and consistency in the diagnosis and treatment of BPH, the Agency for Health Care Policy and Research (AHCPR), an arm of the U.S. Department of Health and Human Services, has collaborated with the American Urological Association to develop guidelines on treatment and nontreatment for both doctors and the public. You can write for a copy at the address listed at the end of this book. Be sure to mark the envelope "BPH."

The American Urological Association Symptom Index

If you have signs of BPH, you'll probably hear of the American Urological Association symptom index at some point during your diagnosis. In a nutshell, the index is a short list of questions that allows your practitioner to assess the severity of your problem. The assessment is then used when determining your course of treatment. The index includes the following questions:

- Over the past month, how often have you had a sensation of not emptying your bladder completely after you have finished urinating?

- Over the past month, how often have you had to urinate again less than two hours after you finished urinating?

- Over the past month, how often have you found you stopped and started again several times when you urinated?

- Over the past month, how often have you found it difficult to postpone urination?

- Over the past month, how often have you had a weak urinary stream?

- Over the past month, how often have you had to strain to begin urination?

> - Over the past month, how often have you typically had to get up to urinate from the time you went to bed a night until the time you got up in the morning?
>
> Using the index, your practitioner will rate your answers on a scale of 1 to 5 and figure your total. The higher your total number, the greater your need for active treatment may be.

If you are unsure whether you require treatment, consider the fact that most men who put off treatment suffer no consequences from the delay. A number of studies indicate that some surgeries can be deferred for years, if not indefinitely, as long as the men prefer, and are able, to live with the symptoms rather than have the surgery to ameliorate them.

A study begun in the 1970s tracked 108 patients who had been advised to have prostate surgery and had refused. Ten years later, 18 of them had finally had surgery to deal with worsening problems, but the other 90, although bothered by their conditions, were still holding out. The 18 who were operated on after 10 years hadn't been hurt by the delay. Those findings, the researchers concluded, indicated that surgery could be postponed in many cases, perhaps indefinitely.

Of course, it all depends on the severity of your symptoms and your willingness to tolerate discomfort. A study comparing the results of watchful waiting with transurethral resection of the prostate (TURP), the most common surgical procedure for BPH, for 550 men in nine Veterans Administration hospitals concluded that TURP was effective for men with moderate symptoms but that watchful waiting was adequate for men whose symptoms were mild, according to John H. Wasson, M.D., an internist specializing in geriatric medicine at Dartmouth Medical School.

If you're considering surgical treatment, be sure your symptoms really are severe and that they're from BPH. As we explain in Chapter 3, many people have urinary problems, and there are indications that many of the men who are operated on for BPH don't actually have the condition. In a 1992 article in the *Journal of Urology,* Edward McGuire, M.D., a urologist at the University of Texas Health Science Center in Houston, said that "we misidentify some 25 to 50 percent of the patients who undergo transurethral resection of the prostate as suffering from obstructive uropathy [a urethra narrowed by BPH] when, in fact, they do not."

Getting a Second Opinion

Already you can see that there are controversies surrounding prostate treatments and when they are appropriate. One valuable tool at your disposal when you're considering your options—which we present in the next section—is the second opinion.

When faced with any sort of serious medical procedure or surgery, you should seek a second opinion. With a prostate condition, getting a second opinion is absolutely vital because of the variety of treatments available and the wide spectrum of opinions held by practitioners in the field.

A second opinion is simply another practitioner's recommendation on your diagnosis and treatment—the opinion of a second, independent health-care practitioner. This and the first opinion can be compared and taken into consideration when you are making a decision about medical care.

While at one time getting a second opinion was considered to be overly cautious and expensive, today many insurers insist that a second opinion be sought before they will cover a procedure. A second opinion is useful because not all doctors agree on medical problems—what they are, how to diagnose them, and how (or even whether) to treat them.

A second opinion is especially important when a trip to the hospital looms. Even a good doctor, convinced that the benefits of surgery outweigh more conservative and less costly treatment, can be eager to rush you into the operating room. A second opinion might confirm the original diagnosis (and perhaps the need for hospitalization), but it could also contradict the first doctor's conclusions and thus precipitate some doubt about the need for hospitalization. You may even require a third, tie-breaking opinion.

But don't limit the search for a second opinion merely to procedures that involve surgery. Many types of therapy—and even diagnostic tests—performed in a hospital are risky or invasive even though not surgical. Ask another doctor for assurance about the need for any procedure that concerns you.

How do you go about getting a second opinion? You should consider finding a doctor for a fair and original second opinion rather than accepting a referral from your practitioner. A lot of second-opinion doctors recommended by first-opinion doctors turn out to be far from impartial. This is true in part because surgeons are the doctors most often asked for second opinions, and they generally recommend surgery over less invasive procedures.

The other, more prevalent problem is that second-opinion doctors may be reluctant to disagree with the friend who recommended them. The truth is that doctors depend on each other for referrals, and too many nonconfirming second opinions may lead to a loss of referrals.

To find a practitioner, check *The Official ABMS Directory of Board-Certified Medical Specialists* in your local library's reference section. In addition, check with your employer's benefits department or ask your insurance company to provide you with a list of physicians it uses for its second-opinion program. A Medicare beneficiary may contact the local Social Security Administration office for a directory of doctors who participate in the Medicare second-opinion program.

Surgical Options

We just mentioned that TURP is the most common surgery performed for BPH. However, it is only one of several surgical options available to treat BPH.

The surgical procedure for BPH is called a prostatectomy—really a partial prostatectomy. In this procedure, new tissue that is the result of BPH is removed from the prostatic capsule; the original prostatic tissue is left intact. The prostatic urethra is also removed but is eventually replaced by normal growth of a new lining that comes down from the bladder.

Prostatectomy can take two different forms: closed and open. A closed operation, the approach increasingly used by surgeons, is done without an incision. An open prostatectomy, the method used historically, requires an abdominal incision.

CLOSED PROSTATECTOMY

There are two kinds of closed operations: **transurethral resection of the prostate (TURP)** and **transurethral incision of the prostate (TUIP).** About 95 percent of all operations for BPH are TURPs, which some urologists call "the gold standard" in BPH treatment, and others describe, more flippantly, as the "Roto-Rooter" of prostatectomies.

In a TURP, the surgeon tunnels through the penis and urethra with a **resectoscope** to resect, or cut, the innermost core of the prostate. The resectoscope, a thin tube about 12 inches in length, contains a light, valves for controlling fluid to irrigate the surgical field, and an electric cutting current or tubular knife blade to cut away tissue. It also has a coagulating electrical current to seal the blood vessels that bleed during the operation.

Starting at the center of the prostatic urethra and working outward, the surgeon removes the obstructing tissue a piece at a time. The pieces of prostate tissue that have been cut away, known as prostate "chips," are carried by the fluid into the bladder and then flushed out through the resectoscope.

The second closed surgical approach to BPH is called the TUIP. A TUIP, or transurethral incision of the prostate, is a more limited surgical procedure than a TURP. A variation on the prostatectomy, a TUIP does not cut away at and flush out the enlarged prostatic tissue. Instead, the surgeon, having tunneled through the urethra, uses the resectoscope to make two deep incisions from a point just inside the bladder neck all the way through the prostate. This has the effect of widening the urinary passage.

OPEN PROSTATECTOMY

The other surgical treatments for BPH are open procedures. There are three kinds of open prostatectomies: the **suprapubic,** the **retropubic,** and the **perineal.** The *-pubic* refers to the pubic bone, and as the names suggest, each of these involves a different anatomical approach to the enlarged prostate.

What to Expect After Transurethral Prostatectomy

After you've undergone a TURP or TUIP procedure, your hospital stay may last anywhere from 3 to 10 days. The length of time depends on your condition, the type of surgery you had done, and how quickly you recover.

During recovery you will have a special catheter, called a Foley catheter, inserted in your urethra. The tube drains urine from the bladder into a collection bag. It will stay in place for the first few days after surgery. In some people the catheter triggers painful spasms right after surgery, but these disappear eventually. Once the catheter is removed a few days later, urine will pass over the incision made during surgery, which may cause discomfort. The pain will lessen as the wound heals. Your urinary stream may seem unusually strong after surgery. You may also have some temporary problems controlling urination after surgery, but long-term incontinence is rare. (We address these risks later in this chapter.)

There may also be blood in your urine after surgery, which is normal. It should disappear by the time you leave the hospital. A few weeks after surgery, the scab within the bladder may loosen and blood may again appear in the urine for a short period. If the bleeding does not stop, if your urine is so red you can't see through it, or if you're in pain, you should contact your doctor.

continues

> You may be given antibiotics before or after surgery to help prevent infection. However, because of concerns that antibiotics are being used too widely and are becoming less effective as a result, some doctors prefer to wait until an infection is actually present before prescribing antibiotics.
>
> Once you're home, you should take it easy for a few weeks. Experts recommend drinking plenty of water (at least eight glasses a day) and eating a healthy diet to prevent constipation, which can strain the bowels. You should also avoid lifting heavy objects and driving or operating machinery. Try not to strain or make any sudden, awkward movements that might tear an incision.

In the suprapubic approach, the surgeon cuts from the navel to the pubic bone and then into the lower abdomen and bladder in order to reach down into the prostatic urethra. There are two types of suprapubic operations: a "blind" approach, in which the prostate remains concealed, and a visual approach, in which the surgeon makes an incision that allows him to see the bladder neck.

In either case, the surgeon uses his index finger to scoop out the BPH tissue. It's possible to do this by touch, since the BPH tissue yields easily, while the true prostate is more resistant.

In the retropubic approach, the surgeon makes the same up-and-down incision used in the suprapubic approach, but instead of opening the bladder, he cleans the area under the pubic bone and exposes the entire surface of the prostate. Then he makes an incision in the prostate and, again using his finger and curved scissors, cleans out the BPH tissue.

In the perineal approach, an incision is made through the perineum, between the anus and scrotum, and the prostate is approached from below.

WEIGHING YOUR OPTIONS

Knowing the differences between the various prostate surgeries is an important part of determining a course of treatment. Yet there's much more than simple definitions involved in how to choose the procedure that's right for you. If you're having surgery for BPH, you'll need to decide whether you want to have a TURP, a TUIP, or an open prostatectomy. A number of factors should go into that decision. You'll want to think about your physical condition, your age, the effectiveness of your options, and the risks and complications associated with them. Most important, you'll need to take into account your own feelings and priorities when weighing your choices.

The Pros and Cons of Closed Prostatectomy

If you're considering a closed prostatectomy, you'll need to decide between a TURP and a TUIP. However, it is really impossible to say how they compare. Because TUIP is so little used, there are virtually no data to go on. Urologists who like

TUIP say it's most appropriate when the enlargement is fairly small. It's also been reported that TUIP has fewer complications, a subject we address below. However, a TUIP leaves the obstructing tissue behind, so some experts believe it may be less effective than a TURP.

Whether a TURP will be effective depends a lot on how bad the condition is in the man being treated. In general, studies show that men who have acute urinary retention or severe obstruction before surgery receive the greatest benefit from a TURP. For example, a study of 388 men in the south of England who underwent TURP during 1988 found that the greatest improvement by far was among men whose problems had been the most severe.

Symptoms that the researchers defined as "obstructive," such as hesitancy and fullness, improved more than "irritative" symptoms like frequency and nocturia. The study reported, however, that more than 70 percent of all the men who underwent the procedure said their symptoms overall had decreased and they felt better.

Some men respond better to a TURP than others partly because some men are bothered more by BPH than others. As a study in Maine in the 1980s found, men with similar BPH symptoms reported considerable differences in how much they were bothered by those symptoms.

Just for your frame of reference: In 1997 the average going rate for a TURP was $7,500, while a TUIP cost an estimated

$4,500. Americans spend at least $2 billion annually for TURP. Because it's a procedure that's performed most often on older men, Medicare pays for most TURPs in the United States. Taking into account all that repeat surgery, prostatectomies are the most common form of major surgery in men over 55 years of age. In 1994 Medicare spent $1 billion to cover 221,000 such operations.

The Pros and Cons of Open Procedures

It's wise to start with your physical condition and overall health when considering your options. In general, men who are older than 70 or in poorer health are advised to have TURPs instead of open prostatectomies because TURPs are physically less demanding.

In particular, men who have prostate cancer as well as BPH should avoid open surgery. When cancer has spread from the true prostate, where it began, into BPH tissue, it's often impossible to separate the two tissues during an open prostatectomy. Attempts to remove the BPH tissue may result in tearing the tough capsule that surrounds the prostate gland.

The recovery times for prostate surgery vary as well. Anything that involves a lot of cutting is likely to involve more postoperative pain and a longer hospital stay than a procedure requiring a small incision or none at all. After a 90-minute TURP under a spinal anesthetic, you're probably going to be walking around within 24 hours and released from the hospital within a few days. With open surgery, you could be hospitalized for as long as 10 days.

Although it may seem that open surgery has few advantages, there are some very important reasons why it might be chosen over a closed procedure. First, most doctors feel that a TURP shouldn't be tried if the prostate is very large: 50 grams or more—more than twice the normal size. However, only about 10 percent of all patients develop a prostate that large.

Second, open surgery also makes sense for men who need additional procedures performed at the same time, typically bladder repairs such as removal of large stones or of diverticula—problems we mention in the previous chapter.

Third, some men have hip problems that make it hard to assume the position required for TURP, which is the standard position for childbirth: flat on your back, with legs spread and elevated.

In addition, a TURP is a somewhat trickier procedure than the open approaches. Prominent urologists agree that if you're not in skilled surgical hands, even if you don't have any of the physical problems cited above, you might want to consider an open prostatectomy. In a later section we discuss complications of both kinds of approaches.

Another benefit of open prostatectomies may be that they are more effective in the long run, according to one widely publicized study. Patients in Denmark, England, and Canada were studied by Noralou Roos, Ph.D., a researcher at the University of Manitoba, in Canada. She found that, eight years after surgery, the number of men undergoing their second prostatectomy (open or closed) was substantially higher after a TURP than after an open prostatectomy. The study, which was published in the *New England Journal of Medicine,* reports that second prostatectomies were between three and six times more common after TURPs.

If you decide on an open procedure, you'll also have to determine which open procedure is best for you. Each of the three open approaches has its drawbacks. In a "blind" suprapubic approach, controlling bleeding after the obstructing prostate tissue has been removed can be a problem; the surgeon can't see the site in order to identify which blood vessels need to be sealed. Recovering from both suprapubic approaches can be quite difficult, because the bladder has been cut and the patient may require two catheters in the bladder for several days to drain the blood and urine.

In the retropubic approach, the exposure of the prostate and bladder neck makes it easy to control bleeding, and recovery is easier. But it can be very hard to expose the prostate in men who are obese or who have a narrow or deep bony pelvis.

The perineal approach, which is the oldest of the surgeries for BPH, has a higher risk of causing impotence because the nerves that control erections are exposed during the procedure. For that reason it's rarely used today.

Risk of Recurrence

It's unfortunate, but true: It is possible for BPH to come back. A prostatectomy, whether open or closed, typically offers only temporary relief from BPH. The reason? The surgery leaves intact the prostate, which is perfectly capable of enlarging a second time. It's commonly said that the benefit of the operation lasts between 15 and 20 years. Since the typical prostatectomy patient is over 65, most men don't live long enough to require a second procedure. Another way of putting the odds is that 10 percent of the men who have the procedure once will ultimately need it again.

Men who had their first surgery at an early age are usually those most likely to need a second prostatectomy. To illustrate that, here's a good example from the front pages of newspapers nationwide. Former President Reagan had his first TURP in 1967, when he was a comparatively young man for the procedure. At the time he was warned he'd probably need another TURP, and right on schedule, 20 years later and at 76 years of age, he was back in the operating room.

Yet, as we said earlier, some men are undergoing prostatectomies within eight years of their first, according to the Roos study. And other studies suggest that the 15-to-20-year figure may be on the rosy side. A study led by John Wennberg, M.D., M.P.H., analyzed the Medicare records of 15,000 men in New England who'd had TURPs. It found that about 20 percent of the men had a repeat TURP within five years, presumably because their symptoms had recurred.

> No one is sure why the reoperation rate is higher for TURP than for open surgery. One theory, offered by Stephen N. Rous, M.D., author of *The Prostate Book,* is that the foreign physicians in the study were not as expert at the operation as those in the United States—hence the higher rate of second TURPs, as well as the greater number of other complications. Without further research, it's hard to know whether the surgeons' skill levels were a critical factor.

Evaluating Mortality Rates

Both open and closed prostatectomies have traditionally been considered very safe procedures, resulting in very few deaths or complications. Various studies report a mortality rate hovering around 1 percent in the first month after either type of procedure—lower for men in their sixties, higher for men in their eighties.

A higher mortality rate was reported by Wennberg, Roos, and other researchers who analyzed claims data for some 4,600 men over the age of 65 who'd had prostatectomies in Manitoba or Maine in the mid-1970s. Three months after the procedure, whether a TURP or an open prostatectomy, the death rate was higher than expected.

But researchers believed one factor behind the differing rates was where the surgery took place. Men who'd had either procedure at smaller hospitals (fewer than 150 beds) were 1.8 times more likely to die in the next three months than men who went to hospitals with 300 beds or more, according to the researchers, whose findings were published in the *Journal of the American Medical Association.*

"The magnitude of the death rate following prostatectomy and its variation by hospital suggest the operation should not be viewed as low-risk or 'minor' surgery," the authors concluded. In other words, the quality of the health-care providers and hospitals was critical.

But which has a higher mortality rate: a TURP or an open prostatectomy? The study we just mentioned implied that TURP and open prostatectomy have about the same risk. But other work by the same researchers suggests that a TURP might actually be riskier. The Roos study we mentioned earlier, which found a higher rate of second prostatectomies after TURPs, indicated that TURPs may be less safe than open prostatectomies. The study reports that men who underwent TURPs had a higher mortality rate during the following five years than those who'd received open prostatectomies.

Even after "risk-adjusting" the data to reflect the fact that open-prostatectomy patients tend to be healthier, the researchers found that men who'd undergone a TURP were 1.5 times more likely to die within five years than were those who'd had open surgery.

The findings of that study—that open surgery is actually safer than a TURP—were hotly disputed. The *New England*

Journal of Medicine, which published the study, editorialized that it "does not provide convincing evidence that open prostatectomy carries less risk than TURP."

No one is sure, if the Roos findings were accurate, why TURP would have a higher mortality rate than open surgery. Roos stated that the "most striking difference in the risk of death"—a relative risk of 2.5 in TURP patients—came from heart attacks. But it's not at all clear why a TURP would lead to a heart attack. British researchers, noting that cardiac output, which is the amount of blood pumped by the heart, falls after a TURP, suggest that the absorption of irrigation fluid that is used to keep the surgical area clear of blood during the procedure may somehow affect the heart and lead to a heart attack. Still, that's only a guess.

A few years later urologists breathed a sigh of relief when John Concato, M.D., at the Yale University School of Medicine concluded, in a study published in the *New England Journal of Medicine* in 1992, that TURPs and open prostatectomies had similar mortality rates five years after the procedure. The reason for any seeming difference, Concato said, was that older, sicker patients underwent TURPs. The same conclusion was reached by authors of a 1995 study from Oxford.

Whether TURP is as safe as open surgery is still a controversial issue in urological circles, and researchers agree that more study is desirable. However, because TURP has virtually supplanted every other surgical approach (as we said earlier,

95 percent of all operations for BPH are TURPs), it's getting harder to analyze the relative merits of TURP over other procedures.

Complicating Factors

You've probably heard that surgery for BPH leads to such complications as impotence, or loss of erection, and incontinence, or loss of urinary control. While it's true that all the surgical approaches to BPH, including TURP, involve some risks in those areas, the risks are not nearly as bad as you might think.

When making your decision about surgery, you should consider the odds that either condition will develop. Short-term incontinence is fairly common, but only a small percentage of the men who have prostatectomies continue to have problems over the long run. As for impotence, it can take up to a year to recover sexual function, but ultimately most men who were able to have erections before the procedure recover that ability. (Erection problems and their treatments are discussed in more detail in Chapter 6.)

It's difficult to give precise numbers because, particularly in the case of sexual function, many men had problems well before they underwent surgery. However, using information gleaned from past studies, the AHCPR estimates the risk for total urinary incontinence to be 1.3 to 2.7 percent for those undergoing TUIP, and 0.68 to 1.4 percent for those having TURP. As for impotence, AHCPR estimates a 3.9 to 24.5 percent risk for TUIP and 3.3 to 34.8 percent for TURP. The risk of total incontinence with open surgery is estimated to be 0.34 to 0.74 percent for open prostatectomies; for impotence, the estimate is 4.7 to 39.2 percent. The range of figures takes into consideration individual characteristics such as age and progression of the disease—your doctor should be able to tell you if you fall into a low-risk or high-risk category for these complications.

A prostatectomy may cause incontinence because of the relationship between the prostate and the urethra. You control urine flow through two mechanisms: the muscles that surround the prostate gland and maintain the tone of the prostatic urethra and bladder neck; and the external urethral sphincter. It's possible for either mechanism to be damaged during a TURP.

Keep in mind that surgery isn't the only cause of either impotence or incontinence. Even if the external, or voluntary, sphincter isn't damaged by the operation, it may already be weakened from disuse. That's because, for months or probably years before the operation, the prostate itself became the main shutoff valve when you urinated. When the external sphincter is damaged, you may have a condition known as **stress incontinence.**

With stress incontinence, you may involuntarily leak urine when increased pressure within your abdomen squeezes down on your bladder. Such pressure can occur when you sneeze, cough, laugh, or exert yourself physically by, say, lifting a heavy weight. It's found most often in women who have given birth vaginally, but it can also affect men after prostate surgery.

The degree of incontinence suffered depends on how much damage is done to either of the mechanisms we described. If the musculature around the prostate is damaged, you can become completely incontinent. However, that's extremely rare after BPH surgery. Stress incontinence, which involves minor losses of urine, is more likely.

Both incontinence and impotence can be treated. Because impotence occurs far more often as a side effect of therapy for prostate cancer, we discuss the condition and various treatments in Chapter 6.

Treating Incontinence

It is true that incontinence is a risk when treating benign prostatic hyperplasia with surgery—one that you'll need to consider when deciding on medical care. Keep in mind, however, that incontinence can be lessened or cured, depending upon how far you want to go with various treatments.

There's a wide range of options, including surgical remedies, medication, continuous catheterization, and external collection devices called condom catheters. Even something as simple as weight loss, if you're obese, may ease your symptoms. There are also many treatments that you can do yourself as soon as your catheter is removed.

Pelvic muscle exercises, called Kegel exercises, are at the top of the list of self-help techniques that can ease incontinence. Although they've been recommended primarily for women after childbirth, they appear to help men too, particularly if the men have mild stress incontinence.

To do these exercises, you must first identify the specific muscles that are responsible for closing the urethra and stopping the flow of urine. If you don't know which ones they are, try tightening your muscles while you're actually urinating. You should practice contracting these muscles repeatedly, for 10 seconds each time, over a period of weeks or months. Just how frequently you need to do the exercises to rebuild muscle strength is disputed; some practitioners recommend "periodic" exercise, while others call for 1,000 contractions a day. You should discuss an exercise regimen with your doctor.

Another self-help method that is widely used is **biofeedback.** It employs electrical monitoring devices, inserted into the rectum, that monitor your movements and give you minute-to-minute information on how well you're controlling your sphincter. One biofeedback study, at the University of Pittsburgh, of men who were incontinent after prostate surgery, reported an 80 percent reduction in leakage. While biofeedback is characterized as self-help, it requires a little outside help from professionals, and that costs time and effort. You'll need to find a therapist who's trained in the technique, and you'll probably need to go to a clinic at least once a week for a few months. You'll need to use the device at home too. Your insurance company can tell you whether it covers such treatments.

If self-help isn't enough to take care of incontinence, other options are available. At the other end of the spectrum is a comparatively elaborate device called an **artificial urinary sphincter**. The device—a **prosthesis** consisting of a balloon, a fluid-filled cuff that encircles the urethra, and a pump implanted in your scrotum—is implanted in a one- to two-hour surgical procedure done using a general anesthetic. The components, which are linked together with tubing, are put into place through two incisions, one below the scrotum and another across the lower abdomen.

To urinate, you squeeze the pump in your scrotum, which forces the fluid out of the cuff around the urethra and into the balloon. As the cuff squeezing the urethra empties, the urine in the bladder is allowed to drain out of the body. After several minutes the fluid in the balloon automatically runs back into the cuff, again preventing urine from leaking from the bladder. The device, which prevents involuntary leakage, is generally recommended for people who suffer from severe incontinence.

According to Rebecca Chalker and Kristene E. Whitmore, authors of *Overcoming Bladder Disorders,* doctors who have implanted the device report that 75 to 85 percent of their patients are satisfied with it. In 10 to 15 percent of the men who have an artificial sphincter, the authors say, "mechanical failures and tissue degeneration in the area of the implants have occurred. Like most mechanical devices, an artificial sphincter may break or wear out after a while and may need to be replaced—so before you decide to get a sphincter implanted, you should be aware that you may need a second surgery to remove or replace it."

For more information, at the back of this book we've listed some groups that specialize in helping people who are incontinent.

Even if a prostatectomy doesn't cause impotence, it does produce something called **dry orgasm,** or **retrograde ejaculation,** in many men. In fact, the AHCPR estimates retrograde ejaculation occurs up to 55 percent of the time in those who have had TUIP and up to 99 percent of the time in TURP patients. In those who have open prostatectomies, the estimate is up to 95 percent. To explain what retrograde ejaculation is, first we'd better describe what happens during a normal orgasm.

During sexual activity sperm from the testicles enter the urethra near the opening of the bladder. Normally, a muscle blocks off the entrance to the bladder, the external sphincter opens, and contracting muscles of the urethra expel the sperm-laden semen through the penis.

During a prostatectomy, however, the bladder neck is frequently enlarged and thus cannot close completely. So when the muscles of the urethra contract, the semen is ejaculated backward through the open internal sphincter and into the bladder. Later the semen gets flushed out in the urine.

If you can't ejaculate semen, you can't reproduce—or at least, not in the tried-and-true way. Fortunately, most men who

Dealing with Incontinence

Incontinence, whether it is temporary or long-term, shouldn't keep a person from living an active life. To help people achieve that goal, a number of products are available to help them cope with urinary problems. These include pads, adult briefs, and bed pads to protect linens and mattresses. Pads are worn under the clothing and are slimmer than briefs; briefs are thicker, but they provide more protection.

When choosing a product, the American Cancer Society recommends that you think about:

- **Comfort.** Does the product feel comfortable when you are standing, sitting, and moving around? How active can you be with the product?

- **Absorbency.** How long will the product provide protection?

- **Bulk.** Is the product noticeable under normal clothing?

- **Availability.** Is it convenient to obtain the product? Which stores carry the item?

- **Cost.** Are incontinence products covered by your insurance?

Another option is self-catheterization, in which you insert a thin tube into the urethra to drain the bladder. The technique is safe, usually painless, and can be taught to you by a physician. Condom catheters—sheaths placed over the penis—and

> compression devices worn on the penis are also options. Talk with your doctor about which choice is right for you. Keep in mind, however, that incontinence products aren't meant to be a permanent solution to urinary problems. Treatment should be sought as well.

undergo prostatectomies already have their families and are well past the age when they want more children. As for the sensation of dry orgasm, many men say it feels peculiar but not unpleasant. It simply takes getting used to. However, if you believe that retrograde ejaculation could be a serious problem for you, some urologists say you should consider an alternative to TURP. TUIP, for example, is less likely to result in this condition.

If you do still want children after a prostatectomy, there are steps you can take. You can try **artificial insemination,** a method widely used in cases of infertility. In a doctor's office, your sperm would be extracted from your urine after retrograde ejaculation. It would then be deposited in your partner's vagina.

Incontinence and retrograde ejaculation aside, another common complication of prostatectomy is urethral stricture, or scarring, which decreases the size of the channel through which urine flows and creates an obstruction as bad as or worse than the problem that led to a TURP in the first place. This generally happens if the resectoscope used in a TURP is too large for the urethra.

About 10 to 15 percent of the men who undergo TURP develop strictures. Usually, a doctor can resolve the problem by stretching the urethra during an office visit.

In a very few cases, the bladder neck gets cut instead of BPH tissue. When it heals, it scars and shrinks so badly that there's only a pinhole opening for urine. When this happens, the patient may need a repeat operation, similar to a TUIP, to widen the bladder neck.

Bacterial infections are not common, but they do happen. Some doctors prescribe preventive antibiotics for several weeks following prostate surgery; others wait to see if infection actually occurs.

One other possible complication is **epididymitis,** an inflammation and enlargement of the epididymis, the sperm-carrying structure we mention in Chapter 1. It can result from infected urine. You also run a slight risk of developing a persistent bacterial infection after prostate surgery from conditions such as incomplete bladder emptying (which may be due to incomplete removal of obstructing BPH tissue) and obstruction of a kidney that has bacteria in it.

Nonsurgical Options

Prostatectomy is not the only option for those with BPH—other alternatives, though less popular, are available. A less invasive procedure for BPH is **balloon urethroplasty,** or **balloon dilatation** of the urethra. It works on the same principle as balloon treatment for coronary arteries. The tissue causing the obstruction isn't removed, just pushed out of the way.

In balloon urethroplasty, a doctor inserts a thin tube with a balloon on its tip into the opening of the penis. He guides it to the narrowed portion of the urethra, where the balloon is inflated. This action compresses the prostate and widens the urethra, easing the flow of urine. The 15-minute procedure can be done in a urologist's office under local anesthesia, though it may take up to four days for a man to resume his regular routine. Short-term complications such as bleeding, infection, and an inability to urinate occur in 2 to 10 percent of patients.

The AHCPR reports the likelihood of improvement with balloon dilatation to be 37 to 76 percent, and the extent of the improvement is rated to be 51 percent. However, this improvement might only be temporary. While men who've had the procedure report that it became much easier initially to urinate, indications are that the symptoms of BPH return fairly soon.

One study found that balloon dilatation and cystoscopy—a diagnostic procedure that isn't designed to relieve symptoms—had about the same effect. Studies at the Mayo Clinic indicate that the effect of balloon urethroplasty may not last beyond a year or two, and only for a limited group of men. Doctors who've worked with the treatment say the best candidates are younger men who have relatively mild symptoms—prostates that aren't terribly enlarged, urinary retention that's not too bad—and who express considerable concern about their ability to maintain erections and to ejaculate.

Balloon urethroplasty could also provide welcome relief for people who are high surgical risks, such as men with advanced prostate cancer and urinary retention or nursing home patients who require catheters.

An alternative to the balloon is **hyperthermia,** a procedure first used with good results to treat obstructions in men with prostate cancer. Also known as **thermotherapy,** it involves the application of heat to the enlarged prostate. There are two approaches, through either the rectum or the urethra, but both combine microwave heating with conductive cooling.

The difference between the two approaches to heat therapy is the way in which the heat is administered. In **transurethral microwave thermotherapy (TUMT),** a modified Foley catheter containing a microwave antenna is inserted through the urethra and heats the tissues deep within the prostate to 45°C (113°F) or higher. Cold water runs through the catheter to provide some comfort and prevent heating up (and possibly shrinking or killing) tissue in the prostatic urethra. The procedure, which takes about an hour, can be carried out in a urologist's office with only local anesthesia.

In transrectal microwave hyperthermia, the water-cooled catheter is placed in the rectum, and the temperature of the prostate tissue is heated to about 43°C (109°F). This one-hour treatment requires no anesthesia, but it involves several more applications than the transurethral approach. It's administered two times weekly over the course of a month or two.

Strangely enough, nobody really knows how the heat works. When the transrectal approach is used, the prostate shrinks very little and there's no sign of the **necrosis,** or tissue death, that would reduce the enlarged gland. It's been suggested that the heat relaxes muscle tissue in the prostate, easing the tightening around the urethra. With transurethral heat therapy, there's definite necrosis of the enlarged prostate, and the obstruction shrinks.

Still, heat therapy is believed to be effective. In fact, the more heat, the more effective it is thought to be. In various studies, both approaches got excellent marks; most of the men who were treated said their urinary problems improved significantly, and urodynamic studies tended to confirm the men's subjective reports.

The procedure is still relatively new. Only in May 1996 did the Food and Drug Administration (FDA) approve the Prostatron, the device for transurethral microwave thermotherapy. Because the equipment just became available, few hospitals are able to offer the treatment. And because the procedure is so new, we don't have much indication of its long-term efficacy. One study at seven medical centers in the United States and Europe reported that 75 percent of men treated with the Prostatron had fewer urinary symptoms, such as urgency, frequency, straining, and intermittent flow. Four years later 50 percent of those men still reported lessened symptoms. The other half, however, required further treatment at some time during those four years. As required by the FDA, studies are continuing on the procedure.

In the meantime, we know there may be some complications with heat therapy, and some men aren't suited for the procedure. Men with greatly enlarged prostates may be poor candidates for hyperthermia, as their glands are hard to reach. For all men, the middle lobe of the prostate is also hard to reach, and that, unfortunately, is usually responsible for the obstruction.

As for complications, occasionally the transrectal approach has resulted temporarily in painful urination or bloody urine. With the transurethral approach, patients often are unable to urinate for up to three days after the procedure. Catheters drain their urine during that time. However, no major complications, such as impotence or retrograde ejaculation, have been reported so far.

One drawback to these devices is that they are quite elaborate, with computer consoles, treatment modules, and ultrasound machines—and price tags to match. Ultimately, however, they could be far more cost-effective than surgery. One estimate put the cost of treatment with the Prostatron at $3,500.

A variation on microwave therapy, radio-wave therapy, known as transurethral needle ablation (TUNA), was approved by the FDA in early 1997. In TUNA, a needle that emits radio waves is inserted through the urethra into the prostate. Again, the heat it produces destroys unwanted prostate tissue. Like TUMT, TUNA costs around $3,500.

One advantage of TUNA is that it is effective on tissue within the middle lobe of the prostate, where TUMT cannot reach. Another advantage is that it usually does not affect urination, meaning a catheter would not be required in the days after treatment.

Another nonsurgical procedure, the expandable wire **stent**, was approved in May of 1996 by the FDA for men in whom standard surgical procedures failed to relieve symptoms of urinary obstruction. A tiny tube, known as the UroLume Endoprosthesis, is implanted into the urethra and expanded to widen the passage and improve urine flow. Gradually, tissue grows over the implant, stabilizing it. In clinical trials, all men reported improved urine flow and improved prostate symptoms. Side effects included dribbling (in about half of all patients), incontinence, pain, blood in the urine, and infection. Some 15 percent of men with stents reported pain with erection and ejaculation, though in most cases this side effect disappeared within six months. Further studies are currently being conducted.

An experimental procedure is **ultrasonic aspiration** of the prostate. Using a device similar to a resectoscope, which is inserted through the urethra, a doctor directs ultrasound vibrations against the enlarged portion of the prostate and "disrupts" the BPH tissue, which is then aspirated, or sucked out, through the urethra.

There's also been an effort to apply **cryosurgery** to BPH. In this treatment, probes are inserted into the prostate through the urethra, and liquid nitrogen is circulated through the probes to freeze and kill the BPH tissue. The tissue is then flushed out through a catheter. While the procedure seems to work, a number of men who've been treated have developed infections and hemorrhaging. Cryosurgery may be better at treating prostate cancer than BPH, as we discuss in the next chapter.

Lasers, which are on the cutting edge in medicine, are being investigated as a possible way to get rid of BPH. In the future we may see **transurethral ultrasound-guided laser-induced prostatectomy**—a procedure with the happy acronym of TULIP—used increasingly as an alternative to surgery.

This is how it works: A laser probe is inserted into the urethra. Using an ultrasound probe in the rectum to direct the laser energy, the doctor uses the beam to superheat and destroy BPH tissue. A week or two later the dead tissue sloughs out though the urethra. A variation known as visual laser ablation of the prostate uses a microtelescope to guide the laser into position.

One study from Stanford University and the Veterans Affairs Medical Center in Palo Alto, California, reported that 85 to 90 percent of men treated with the laser surgery were able to urinate more easily after the procedure. The procedure reportedly results in little or no bleeding, and little anesthesia is required. None of the men in the study reported incontinence, and researchers say the complication is very unlikely when the procedure is done correctly. However, laser therapy is still in its experimental stages.

Medications

Surgery aside, medications are available to treat BPH. There's been a lot of talk lately about the "prostate pill." It's clearly an idea whose time has come, but the pill itself has yet to be developed. That's the bad news. The good news is that, after all these years, there are drugs in the pipeline that may eventually offer a real alternative to surgery.

There are two major categories of prostate drugs. The first is **antihypertensives,** which have the effect of relaxing the smooth muscle tissue in the prostate and bladder neck, easing constriction of the urethra. These are also known as alpha-adrenergic blockers.

The second category is 5-alpha-reductase inhibitors. They inhibit the production of DHT, which, as we discuss in Chapter 3, seems to be responsible for prostate enlargement.

Scientists are also investigating a third drug category: aromatase inhibitors. The enzyme **aromatase** converts testosterone into the form of estrogen that is found in all men. It may contribute to BPH in older men who, as part of the normal aging process, develop higher amounts of estrogen relative to testosterone. Aromatase drugs, such as atamestane, block this action. Research in this category, however, is in the early stages.

You may recognize antihypertensives as drugs used for people with high blood pressure. In fact, their potential for treating BPH was first noticed when it was reported in 1978 that one of the drugs, prazosin (brand name Minipress, manufactured by Pfizer), resulted in urinary incontinence in women who were being treated for hypertension. Since then, the Food and Drug Administration has approved two antihypertensives for treating BPH: terazosin (brand name Hytrin, manufactured by Abbott) and doxazosin (brand name Cardura, manufactured by Pfizer). Terazosin runs about $575 per year, and doxazosin costs about $450 annually.

Antihypertensives have been shown to be effective in treating BPH. A three-year study of terazosin, published in *Urology* in 1995, found that, within a few months of starting the drug, most patients reported their symptoms were considerably better—specifically, their urinary flow rates were much higher.

Like most drugs, antihypertensives have a well-established list of adverse reactions and side effects, and obviously there's some trepidation about their regular use by people whose blood pressure is normal. About 20 percent of patients dropped out of the terazosin study, for example, because the drug's side effects—such as dizziness, fatigue, and weakness—were too severe. On the plus side, the researchers noted that terazosin lowered blood pressure primarily in men who were hypertensive but not in those whose blood pressure was normal. Side effects can be minimized by taking antihypertensives at bedtime or after a substantial meal. Many of the side effects subside after a few days or weeks of drug therapy.

Another type of drug approved specifically to treat BPH is finasteride, better known as Proscar, the name under which it's being marketed by Merck. The FDA approved Proscar in mid-1992. It is in the second category of drugs we mentioned earlier: a new family of agents called 5-alpha-reductase inhibitors, which work by blocking the conversion of testosterone into DHT. We mention the 5-alpha-reductase enzyme in Chapter 3.

Proscar is somewhat effective against BPH. It seems to be especially effective in shrinking enlarged prostates and keeping them shrunk. But many urologists note that it's less effective at symptom relief. In 12-month clinical trials, Merck found that urine flow increased and other symptoms improved in less than half of the men taking the drug.

Other research has been aimed at figuring out whether men on finasteride are less likely to need BPH surgery or suffer urinary retention than men not taking the drug. A 1998 study (funded, incidentally, by the drug manufacturer and conducted by authors with financial ties to that company) found that finasteride was effective, reducing the rate of urinary retention by 57 percent and the need for prostatectomy by 55 percent.

The statistics certainly sound impressive. But critics point out that symptoms often don't progress in men with BPH and that the drug is expensive (more than $800 per year). In fact, only 13 percent of men in the four-year study who weren't taking the drug ended up having urinary retention and having surgery. One editorial in the *New England Journal of Medicine* points out that, over a four-year period, only 5 out of each 100 men (who'll each shell out some $3,200) will avoid surgery because of the drug.

"For patients with advanced disease, surgery remains the treatment of choice," says Reginald Bruskewitz, M.D., of the University of Wisconsin Clinical Science Center. "However, Proscar offers a medical option for many patients."

You might expect Proscar to cause impotence and other complications because it tampers with DHT levels. Circulating testosterone remains high, however, so there's usually no effect on a man's ability to have erections. In its clinical trials, Merck found that 3.7 percent of the subjects became impotent, 3.3 percent reported decreased libido, and 2.8 percent ejaculated less semen when they had orgasms. Some men also reported a general physical weakness.

Gynecomastia, enlargement of the male breast, may also be a side effect of Proscar. In fact, the FDA says it is the most frequently reported adverse effect of the drug. Researchers surmise that Proscar may increase the ratio of estrogen to androgen in the body through its conversion of dihydrotestosterone, causing breast tissue to grow. There is some concern that use of the drug may be associated with the development of breast cancer in men, and long-term studies on the possibility are currently underway.

Another side effect, one perhaps of greater immediate concern to the medical community, is that finasteride lowers serum concentrations of prostate-specific antigen by up to 50 percent. Since, as we discuss in the previous chapter, the PSA test is being used increasingly to screen for prostate cancer, there's a lot of concern that Proscar can make it difficult to detect cancer.

Merck has said that doctors can easily factor in Proscar's impact on PSA levels when they test for prostate cancer. Urological experts say they don't know whether that's really feasible, however. Nor do they know whether men who develop prostate cancer will have elevated PSA levels if they're taking Proscar.

This doesn't mean that Proscar increases the risk of prostate cancer. In fact, just the opposite may be true. Men with the genetic 5-alpha-reductase deficiency (see Chapter 3) don't often get prostate cancer. As we said earlier, Proscar is a 5-alpha-reductase inhibitor. Early studies being conducted by the National Cancer Institute have found that finasteride, at certain dosages, reduced prostate cancer incidence in rats. It is not yet known, however, if the drug will do the same in humans.

So far, Proscar seems relatively safe for men. But it may be quite dangerous for women! Animal studies have shown that Proscar can harm male fetuses. So although the drug is present in male semen only in minute amounts, women who are or may become pregnant should avoid being exposed to the semen of men taking Proscar. That means no sexual relations—at least not without the use of condoms—with women of childbearing age. In addition, women who are or may become pregnant should avoid handling crushed tablets of Proscar so that they will not absorb the drug through their skin.

Proscar, which is to be taken daily in a 5-milligram dose, costs users about $825 a year. That's a bitter pill to swallow, especially if you've got to take it daily for the rest of your life. Once men stop taking finasteride, serum DHT returns to its previous level within two weeks, and BPH symptoms come back.

Whether the cost of Proscar will be covered by insurance depends on your specific health insurance or managed care plan and the formulary (list of prescription medications) it's willing to cover. The only way you're going to know for sure is to read the schedule of benefits, which tells you what is covered and what is not. If this doesn't answer your question, then ask your plan's marketing representative. If the answer is no, you might ask your primary care physician to intervene on your behalf. If she can attest that the medication will be effective in your case, the plan may reconsider and cover it.

There has been a lot of controversy over which drug is better: the antihypertensive (Hytrin) or finasteride (Proscar). That's a highly contentious issue right now, with Proscar and Hytrin competing aggressively in the marketplace.

Recently Hytrin scored a coup, with the preliminary results of a study of 1,130 men in Veterans Administration hospitals who received either Proscar, Hytrin, both, or a placebo. Researchers reported that, while Proscar shrank the prostate 20 percent, it did little to relieve prostate symptoms after a year of use. In fact, Proscar did no better than a placebo at easing urinary problems. Hytrin, on the other hand, did improve symptoms. The combination of drugs improved symptoms no more than Hytrin used alone did.

Those findings are inconsistent with past research on Proscar. Merck counters that the study was too short-term and that it wasn't used on men with extremely enlarged prostates, where Proscar is most effective. That reasoning is backed up by a September 1996 analysis published in *Urology*, which reported that finasteride works better than a placebo but only in men with larger prostates. Terazosin is thought to work best on men with mildly enlarged prostates.

Still, it's hard to say at this point which one you should take. More information will be forthcoming from comparative studies of finasteride and the two antihypertensives.

In the meantime, researchers at the University of Texas Southwestern Medical Center, who recently concluded their own study of terazosin, suggested that—because it either works or doesn't work within a few weeks—it's a logical first choice before trying finasteride or surgery. On the other hand, finasteride may be the first choice for men with greatly enlarged prostates.

There's also interest in the medical community in combining the two drugs. Finasteride has its greatest effect on the glandular parts of the prostate, while the muscle relaxants act mainly on the prostate's muscle and connective tissue. So doctors feel there might be potential in a drug combination that relaxes the prostate muscle while shrinking the prostatic tissue.

At this point, both drug types are pretty problematic, and insiders agree that we're seeing just the first wave of medical therapy for BPH. Merck is already working on a more potent "son of Proscar."

The newest drug on the prostate scene works in a way similar to terazosin but more selectively, to produce fewer side effects. Flomax (tamsulosin HCl), developed by Boehringer Ingelheim Pharmaceuticals, is a prostate-selective alpha$_{1A}$-adrenoreceptor agonist—a mouthful, that's for sure. But what the drug does is simpler than its name: It works by blocking only the specific receptors around the bladder neck and prostate, which results in relaxation of the tissues and improved urinary flow. Because the drug doesn't affect blood vessels, the manufacturer says, it does not alter blood pressure, as a true antihypertensive does. Flomax also reportedly works faster than nonselective alpha-blockers—about a week after dosing begins, rather than a month. Reported side effects for Flomax include dizziness, infection, abnormal ejaculation, rhinitis, and a risk of syncope (fainting).

At a Glance: BPH Medications

Drug Name	Class	How It Works
terazosin (Hytrin); doxazosin (Cardura)	antihypertensives (also called alpha-adrenergic blockers)	Relaxes the smooth tissue in the neck, prostate and the bladder easing the pressure on the constricted urethra and improving urine flow. May affect blood pressure.
finasteride (Proscar)	5-alpha-reductase inhibitors	Inhibits production of dihydrotestosterone, a form of testosterone that may contribute to BPH
tamsulosin HCI (Flomax)	prostate-selective alpha$_{1A}$-adrenoreceptor agonist	Blocks specific receptors in the prostate and bladder neck to relax tissue and improve urine flow. Does not affect blood pressure.

There are other drugs available that treat BPH through **hormonal therapy,** that is, by reducing levels of testosterone. However, you may not want to take them. Consider the results of a small study at the Johns Hopkins University Medical School. The research looked at **nafarelin acetate,** a hormone blocker that inhibits the production of testosterone. After four months, the subjects' prostates had shrunk by one-fourth, and most of the men reported that their urinary problems had improved. All nine men in the study became temporarily impotent, however. (A tenth subject withdrew after two months, claiming that the loss of libido and drive had hurt his business performance!)

Six months after the medication was stopped, both the men's prostate size and their testosterone levels had returned to the point they were at before treatment. The researchers concluded that the treatment would be appropriate only for a select group of men who couldn't tolerate surgery.

The same problems occurred with estrogen therapy. While it's true that estrogens shrink the prostate enough to relieve symptoms, they also lead to impotence and enlarged, tender breasts.

Self-Care for BPH

Whether you're being treated with medications, thinking of surgery, or practicing watchful waiting, there are methods you can use yourself to treat the enlargement, or at least alleviate prostate symptoms.

- Cut down on fluids in the evening, especially alcohol and caffeine, which stimulate urination

The Power of Placebos

Unlike a lot of medical conditions, BPH is a condition to which men have a highly subjective response. And despite tests such as urodynamic studies, the success of the treatment is difficult to quantify. Often there's a big difference between the symptoms reported by the men themselves and the clinical evidence, such as the data from urodynamic studies, reported by their doctors.

It's interesting to note that, in clinical trials of various treatments for BPH, researchers report a strong placebo effect: People who received nothing more than a placebo, an inactive substance used as a control in an experiment, often reported a significant improvement in symptoms.

Strangely enough, research shows that even a placebo can be effective in cases of mild BPH. The Proscar Safety Plus Efficacy Canadian Two-Year (PROSPECT) study from Ontario, in its research of finasteride, also noticed improved symptoms in men who were unknowingly taking placebos. Even stranger: More than 80 percent of the men taking placebos complained of side effects, such as impotence and decreased libido, that they attributed to the inactive substance.

- Urinate frequently. If you overtax your bladder, you'll only aggravate the symptoms.

- Take your time urinating. Allow several minutes to empty the bladder as completely as possible.

- Be aware that certain prescription drugs can aggravate urinary problems. These include some antispasmodics, including oral bronchodilators, diuretics, tranquilizers, and antidepressants. If you're currently taking such medication and you're at an age when you're likely to develop BPH or already have symptoms, you might want to ask your doctor about reducing the dosage or switching to another drug. There are also some over-the-counter cold remedies, such as antihistamines and decongestants, that can worsen a urinary condition.

- Think about zinc. As we discuss in Chapter 2, many people, both in and outside the medical profession, believe that zinc promotes a healthy prostate. Irving M. Bush, M.D., a urologist at the Chicago Medical School, has put some people on zinc therapy for 20 years and says they seem to need prostate surgery far less often than the norm. He believes that zinc therapy is effective for BPH if it's begun when the prostate first starts to enlarge. The zinc in the body, in his view, keeps the prostate's glandular tissue from enlarging in order to produce more zinc. Bush offers some patients a combination of zinc and muscle relaxants.

- Try saw palmetto. Saw palmetto is an herbal remedy that is thought to be helpful in treating BPH. Made from the berry of a tree found in the southeastern United States, saw palmetto has been found to work better than a placebo in scientific studies on BPH treatments.

The studies, which were done in Italy and France, found that men who took 320 milligrams of saw palmetto daily reported one less nighttime trip to the bathroom than men taking a placebo. Those men using saw palmetto also reported easier, less painful urination and said they could empty their bladders more completely than before. Researchers warn, however, that these studies lasted only a few months and didn't use conclusive questionnaires to evaluate symptoms. As a result, the studies don't necessarily prove the benefits of saw palmetto. In addition, saw palmetto is sold as a supplement, meaning it has not been tested for safety; talk with your doctor about using it to help your problem.

Finally, if you decide to try saw palmetto, look for packages labeled "standardized to 85 percent to 95 percent fatty acids"—the potency that was used in the studies.

Consider other alternatives. Homeopathy offers another self-care option—a combination of three of the amino acids (glycine, alanine, and glutamate) in a daily dosage of several grams. In addition, some people say their symptoms have been eased by lecithin, as well as by calcium and magnesium tablets, all of which are available from pharmacists and health food shops. Certain medicinal herbs, such as *Pygeum africanum* and nettles, have also been found helpful by some. However, there have been no good studies on these treatments to date.

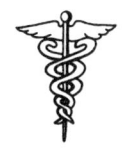

CHAPTER 5

Understanding Prostate Cancer

TALK OF PROSTATE CANCER—OR ANY TYPE OF CANCER, FOR THAT matter—often has an aura of fear and death, bolstered by daunting statistics and concerns about complications such as impotence and incontinence.

There is no denying that prostate cancer is serious. It is important, however, to understand that cancer, especially prostate cancer, is not an automatic death sentence. In fact, the reality of prostate cancer is quite the contrary: Prostatic cancer is generally a very slow-growing malignancy, and the vast majority of these cancers grow so slowly that they never become a threat to life. Hence the common statement that "most men die *with* prostate cancer, not of it."

Concerns about urinary and sexual function are well-founded too, but these complications are probably not as common as you might think—and new technologies are rapidly developing to help avoid them altogether.

In the following pages, we give you information to help dispel that negative aura and get a handle on prostate cancer and its diagnosis. In Chapter 6, there is a thorough discussion of treatment options. Let's start with some facts about the disease itself.

What Is Prostate Cancer?

Cancer of the prostate is almost always a primary cancer, meaning that it originates in the prostate rather than traveling there from another part of the body. Typically, it begins in the outer part of the prostate. As the tumor grows, it may spread to the inner part of the prostate. Like other cancers, prostate cancer can then **metastasize**, or spread, to other parts of the body. If they are not stopped, cancerous cells will continue to multiply, crowding out healthy cells and interfering with the normal functions of the body.

Until quite recently, well-known men who developed prostate cancer declined to go public. Although Cornelius Ryan, author of such bestsellers as *A Bridge Too Far*, wrote a book about his experience with prostate cancer, it's noteworthy that it was called *A Private Battle* (and that it was published posthumously).

These days, however, prominent men such as financier Michael Milkin, politician Bob Dole, and retired general

Norman Schwarzkopf are announcing that they're being treated for the disease, and it has been given as the cause of death in obituaries for entertainment mogul Steve Ross, rock musician Frank Zappa, and French president François Mitterand, among others.

As more men acknowledge their experience with prostate cancer, awareness about the disease and its consequences is increasing. At one time cancer—especially prostate cancer—was a taboo subject among men, who are often reluctant to talk about their personal health in any case. But thanks to prostate cancer's growing public image, more men are realizing the importance of being screened for the condition. The increased attention also means more research money is being spent to develop new procedures and treatments to handle the disease. What's more, men with the disease are enjoying an increased variety of informational resources and support groups as dialogue about prostate cancer becomes public.

But prostate cancer's newfound popularity has its downside too. Because greater numbers of men are now being screened, more men will face false-positive results—that is, being told they have cancer when they actually don't. And men with prostate cancer (which, as you'll remember, grows very slowly) may be subjected to treatments they don't really need. Some of this controversy is reflected by the statistics behind prostate cancer, which we explain next.

> ## Reluctant Patients
>
> How long has it been since you visited the doctor for a routine physical? If you're like most men, it's been a long time. Men are notorious for avoiding their doctors, especially for regular examinations. Instead, many men wait until they're having a health crisis before seeking care—a dangerous gamble considering that many conditions, including prostate cancer, often don't cause symptoms until they have progressed to a serious stage.
>
> Men make a reported 150 million fewer visits to physicians than women do. One recent survey of 1,500 physicians by the Men's Health Network showed that doctors believe that, compared with women, men have more trouble discussing health concerns (especially sexual concerns), are less likely to seek medical attention for complaints, are more likely to delay treatment until a condition worsens, and are less likely to stick to any prescribed treatment plans.
>
> Why don't men go to the doctor? Well, some may feel that they have no reason to visit a doctor on a regular basis and may have a physical only when it's required, perhaps for a sport. Others may be hesitant or embarrassed to talk about their health concerns with a doctor. Active, healthy men may feel they don't need to have regular exams, or they might believe they're too busy to waste time or money on preventive care. Unfortunately, men also tend to put off care when they have serious symptoms,

> shrugging off health problems as unimportant or perhaps postponing care because they're afraid of what the diagnosis might be. They may also be afraid of what the doctor will recommend—lose weight, cut back on salt, quit smoking, quit drinking.

Incidence of Prostate Cancer

In hard numbers, approximately one in every five American men will be diagnosed with prostate cancer during his lifetime. (A woman's lifetime risk of developing breast cancer is one in eight.) In 1998, estimates the American Cancer Society (ACS), prostate cancer will account for 184,500 new cases and 39,200 deaths in the United States. Though this is more than double the number of new cases in 1990, the incidence of prostate cancer stabilized in 1994.

For American men, prostate cancer is the most common type of cancer, excluding skin cancers. And, after lung cancer, it's the main cause of cancer deaths in men. (Admittedly, it's a distant second: Lung cancer claims some 93,000 lives each year.)

The incidence of prostate cancer reached its peak in 1992, when the rate was 186 per 100,000 for Caucasian men and 247 per 100,000 for African American men. Between 1992 and 1993, however, the number of new cases of prostate cancer dropped by 16 percent in Caucasian men and stabilized in African Americans.

The number of new cases in older men of both races declined by 17, to 29 percent.

What does this statistical roller coaster mean? First, let's look at the increase. There are several reasons behind the greater number of prostate cancer cases diagnosed. One obvious explanation is the aging of the population: The incidence of prostate cancer increases with age, and there are currently more people in the United States over age 65 than ever before.

That aside, some researchers at the National Cancer Institute (NCI), who have analyzed mortality trends and laboratory studies of certain prostate tumors, say that part of the initial increase could have been more than statistical, reflecting real changes in the risk of prostatic cancer. But nobody knows why prostate cancer should have been on the rise, except that overall cancer incidence is rising, according to the NCI.

Much of the increase could be attributed to changes in medical practice. One important factor is the growing number of prostatectomies—operations to reduce enlarged prostates. Routine analysis of prostatic tissue removed during the surgery allows doctors to detect prostate cancer at a very early stage, and that adds to the statistics.

Another important factor is the increased screening for prostate cancer, particularly with the highly sensitive prostate-specific antigen (PSA) test. As the disease assumed a much higher profile in the early 1990s, greater numbers of men underwent screening. More cases were diagnosed, raising incidence rates.

Within the past few years, however, some controversies—which we discuss later in this chapter—began to overshadow prostate screening, causing its value to be called into question. As a result, researchers speculate, fewer men are undergoing screening now than in recent years. Some experts also think that the surge in prostate cancer cases could be attributed to the introduction of the PSA screening test. Now that the test has been available for a few years, they say, many of the men with prostate cancer have been diagnosed already, decreasing the rate of new cases. These factors may account for the recent stabilization and decline of cancer rates.

Causes of Prostate Cancer

We've already alluded to some of the factors—such as age—that may increase cancer risk. But before we talk about risks, let's look at the actual causes of prostate cancer. That's a little difficult to do: Exactly what triggers prostate cancer is somewhat of a mystery, although researchers do have some leads. Both epidemiological studies and laboratory research have shown a clear connection between prostate cancer and androgens, or male hormones, especially testosterone.

Research has also suggested a connection between a high-fat diet and high levels of testosterone. Some researchers believe that the fat in foods raises the levels of both testosterone and certain estrogens, which stimulate the prostate to grow, along with any cancer cells the prostate may harbor. A 1996 National Cancer Institute study, in fact, found that men on high-fat, low-fiber diets have testosterone levels that are 13 to 15 percent higher than men on low-fat, high-fiber diets.

Men who have higher testosterone levels seem to have a higher rate of prostate cancer. African Americans, for example, have slightly higher levels of testosterone than Caucasian men. Interestingly, autopsy studies have found that men around the world have a similar incidence of latent carcinoma, or slow-growing microscopic cancers. But in countries where people eat more fat and therefore have higher testosterone levels, these tumors are likely to blossom into full-blown cancer, which is more aggressive—meaning that it spreads and is difficult to cure.

Some men who develop prostate cancer undergo therapy in which their testosterone is removed, either surgically (through removal of the testes) or through hormonal therapy. As a rule, their tumors regress for months or even years. Although the testosterone is gone, eventually the tumors do recur. No one fully understands how testosterone can lead to prostatic cancer or how tumors can recur without it.

Risk Factors for Prostate Cancer

The main risk factor for prostate cancer is age. The older you are, the greater your chances of developing prostate cancer. That one-in-five incidence is for men throughout their lives; it's a rarity in young men, and risk rises steadily with age. More than 80 percent of prostate tumors are diagnosed in men age 65 or older. Autopsy studies have found evidence of prostate cancer in 70 percent of men who were age 80 or older who died of unrelated causes.

There are other risk factors that make some men more likely to get prostate cancer than others. Much like female breast cancer, prostate cancer runs in families. The American Medical Association has estimated that a man whose father or brother had prostate cancer—particularly if the relative was under age 65—has about twice the usual risk of a man his age. NCI's Division of Cancer Prevention and Control has said epidemiological data—statistics on the incidence of disease—show that men who have more than one relative with prostate cancer may have up to six times the average risk. On the whole, studies show that prostate cancer in men with a family history of the disease tends to be aggressive and often difficult to cure.

The other high-risk group is African American men. According to the ACS, they have the highest rate of prostate cancer in the world. They also have double the average mortality rate for men with prostate cancer, though that statistic may reflect their access to medical care rather than physiological factors.

Some researchers think, however, that race isn't nearly as critical a factor as diet. H. Ballentine Carter, M.D., of the Johns Hopkins University School of Medicine, in Baltimore, cites epidemiological data indicating that black men living in Africa

> ### Age and Prostate Cancer Risk
>
> How does your risk of prostate cancer change as you age? Check out these statistics from the American Cancer Society:
>
> | Age | Percent | Risk |
> | --- | --- | --- |
> | Birth to 39 | 1.68 | 1 in 60 |
> | 40 to 59 | 1.74 | 1 in 57 |
> | 60 to 79 | 16.40 | 1 in 6 |
> | Birth to death | 18.85 | 1 in 5 |

have among the lowest rates of prostate cancer in the world, but when they immigrate to the United States, their risk of developing prostate cancer increases tenfold. There are similar findings about Asians who immigrate to this country and abandon their traditional low-fat diets.

A number of epidemiological studies suggest a connection between prostate cancer and diet. The main culprit is fat, especially animal fat. A number of studies show that men who eat large amounts of animal fat have significantly higher rates of prostate cancer than men who eat relatively little animal fat. There's also evidence that men who eat a lot of animal fat develop a form of prostate cancer that spreads faster and is more difficult to cure. As we said before, some researchers believe that a high-fat diet raises testosterone levels and encourages prostate and prostate cancer growth.

A 1994 study at Loma Linda University, in California, for example, found that male Seventh-Day Adventists who ate a diet high in fatty foods (such as meat, cheese, and eggs) were 3.5 times more likely to have fatal prostate cancer than Adventist men who didn't eat those foods very often. (Adventists tend to be vegetarians.) Other studies point to an increased risk for heavy milk drinkers, especially when it's whole milk.

In fact, another study suggested that switching to a low-fat diet may slow the growth of prostate cancer. The study, by researchers at Memorial Sloan-Kettering Cancer Center in New York, showed that tumor growth could be stymied in laboratory mice by halving their intake of fat, to 21 percent or less of daily calories.

Another risk factor for prostate cancer may be birth weight. In a study of 50-year-old men, Swedish researchers found that the incidence of prostate cancer was significantly higher among men who weighed more than 9.3 pounds at birth.

Other proposed risk factors for prostate cancer include a history of sexually transmitted disease and multiple sex partners. In 1997, researchers from the National Cancer Institute reported finding a preliminary link between the human papillomavirus (HPV), associated with sexually transmitted genital warts, and an increased risk of prostate cancer. However, further studies are needed to confirm the link.

Vasectomy and Prostate Cancer

There has been some speculation that a **vasectomy**, the contraceptive procedure in which the vas deferens are cut and sealed off, can lead to prostate cancer. A number of published reports have suggested that a vasectomy slightly increases the risk, while others have found no higher risk in men who have undergone the procedure. According to a May 2, 1995, *Journal of the National Cancer Institute* article, researchers failed to find an association between vasectomy and prostate cancer when looking at men in the United States and Canada. A later study (conducted by the same researchers who in 1993 reported a correlation between vasectomy and prostate cancer) found that there is little support for an association between the two.

Most recently, Spanish researchers analyzed 14 studies on the relationship between vasectomy and prostate cancer. While six of the studies showed a link between the two, the researchers reported they were flawed because the studies failed to take into account other factors that might have affected vasectomy risk (*Fertility and Sterility*, August 1998). As a result, the researchers concluded, there is no good evidence to support an association between cancer and the contraceptive procedure.

An editorial from physicians from the Centers for Disease Control and Prevention that accompanied the study said that "there is little biologic plausibility for an effect of vasectomy on risk of

> prostate cancer, with the arguments for a beneficial effect as strong as those for a harmful effect."
>
> The American Urological Association, the American Cancer Society, and the National Institutes of Health have all issued statements saying that the evidence of any connection between vasectomy and prostate cancer is very weak. Despite this assurance, however, some practitioners are not convinced. A 1996 nationwide survey showed that 27 percent of urologists report that they routinely screen men who have had vasectomies earlier than men who have not undergone the procedure.

Prostate cancer may occur in men who have had a prostatectomy for BPH, though a man's cancer risk isn't increased by the procedure. As we discuss in detail in Chapter 4, a partial prostatectomy for BPH removes the new tissue but leaves the original prostate intact. So, unfortunately, it's as capable of developing cancer as a prostate that's never been touched.

Preventing and Slowing Prostate Cancer

Unfortunately, we know very little about ways to prevent prostate cancer. Of course, there may be some steps you can take to lower your prostate cancer risk. Although you can't change your genetic background or family history of the disease, you can alter your diet and eat more low-fat, high-fiber foods. In addition, practicing safe sex might help reduce your risk by preventing the sexually transmitted diseases that some experts associate with prostate cancer.

There is also speculation about foods that might fight prostate cancer. Some researchers say there's no apparent link between fruits and vegetables that are rich in vitamins A and C and a lower incidence of prostate cancer.

But other studies suggest that a diet of grains, legumes, soy protein, fruits, and vegetables can help prevent prostate cancer. A study of some 750 men by Roswell Park Memorial Institute, in Buffalo, New York, found that a diet high in **beta carotene** seemed to lower the risk for men under age 69 (but didn't affect older men). Beta carotene is found in dark green leafy vegetables such as broccoli and spinach and in deep yellow and orange vegetables and fruits such as carrots and cantaloupe, as well as in vitamin supplements.

However, a study by Harvard researcher Edward Giovannucci, M.D., reported in the *Journal of the National Cancer Institute,* found that the only vegetable that reduced the risk of prostate cancer was the tomato. The study found far lower rates among men who ate at least 10 servings a week of tomato-based foods such as tomatoes, tomato sauce, tomato juice, and pizza. Cooked was better than raw. The benefit is attributed to lycopene, the **carotenoid** that makes tomatoes red.

And while intake of selenium, a mineral antioxidant, has not been shown to have a consistent relationship with prostate cancer, it is a promising possibility. One study shows a 63 percent decrease in the incidence of the disease among men taking selenium supplements. And a 1998 Harvard study found that men with the highest intakes of selenium had a significantly lower risk of prostate cancer than those who had the lowest intakes of the mineral. Additional studies are necessary to confirm this conclusion. Selenium can be found in broccoli, mushrooms, cabbage, celery, cucumbers, onions, garlic, radishes, brewer's yeast, grains, fish, and organ meats such as liver.

Lately some researchers have hypothesized that vitamin D may also be effective against prostate cancer. It's found in vitamin D–enriched milk, fish-liver oil, salmon, tuna, sardines, egg yolks, and margarine and in vitamin supplements. Of course, the major source of vitamin D is sunlight.

This hypothesis has led researchers to consider whether sunlight can fight prostate cancer. While this possibility is still only a hunch, it is an interesting one at that. Published in 1992, a study by researchers at the University of North Carolina at Chapel Hill found that the rate of death from prostate cancer in the United States was significantly lower in the sun-baked South than in the North. The only explanation the researchers had was that people in the South get more UV light, or ultraviolet radiation.

Of course, while UV exposure might decrease your risk of prostate cancer, researchers say it can also boost your risk of skin cancer. Nonetheless, some experts recommend 15 minutes of sun exposure daily to get the benefits of vitamin D. The time frame, they say, is long enough to trigger production of the vitamin but too short to cause skin damage in most people.

Vitamin E may help fight prostate cancer too. The Alpha-Tocopherol, Beta Carotene Cancer Prevention Study, a Finnish study published in the April 14, 1994, *New England Journal of Medicine,* failed to find a link between vitamin E and lung cancer, but—surprise!—it did indicate that the vitamin may reduce the risk of prostate cancer by 34 percent. Almonds, asparagus, duck, goose, kale, spinach, prunes, and sunflower seeds are among the foods that can provide 20 percent or more of your RDA of vitamin E in a 3.5-ounce serving.

Other environmental factors may play a role as well. A recent study found that farmers exposed to herbicides were more than twice as likely to develop prostate cancer as farmers who used no herbicides. The study, of 145,000 farmers in Canada, is the first major research connection between herbicides and prostate cancer. However, since the researchers relied on census data, it could be that other factors, such as diet, led to the different rates of prostate cancer.

As for occupational exposure, studies show that men who do welding or electroplating or who make batteries, and are thus exposed to the metal cadmium, may have a higher risk of getting prostate cancer. A different group—workers in the rubber industry—also seem to be at risk.

Lifestyle factors, such as promiscuity, have also been considered by researchers as risk factors for prostate cancer. There's been speculation that untreated sexually transmitted diseases or cigarette smoking may also increase risk. But no factor has been linked to prostate cancer the way diet has.

Regular exercise has been shown to reduce the risk of prostate cancer. Data from nearly 18,000 men in the Harvard Alumni Health Study over a 15-year period strongly suggest that a consistent exercise regimen over many years may lessen the risk of developing prostate cancer. While 419 men developed prostate cancer, only one case was found among men who described themselves as highly active in 1962 or 1966 and again in 1977.

It's not clear why exercise seems to help. One possible explanation is that increased physical activity may lower the level of testosterone, a primary suspect for prostate cancer. Of course, exercise can also help you control your weight, and that may be a factor in prostate cancer mortality. The Adventist study showed that obese men were 2.5 times more likely to have fatal prostate cancer than men closer to their desirable weight.

At this point, there are no drugs that can prevent prostate cancer. The drug finasteride (manufactured by Merck under the brand name Proscar), however, lowers levels of dihydrotestosterone

(DHT), a hormone that is thought to be a culprit in promoting prostate cancer. For that reason, the National Cancer Institute is running a prostate cancer prevention trial to evaluate the drug's effect on men at high risk for prostate cancer. Proscar must be prescribed by a physician and is now used to treat BPH. More information on Proscar appears in Chapter 4.

Symptoms of Prostate Cancer

Unfortunately, most prostate cancers are "silent," which is to say they don't cause noticeable symptoms or problems for months or even years. The cancer must grow fairly large before it presses on the urethra and causes trouble with urination. Symptoms of more advanced prostate cancer include blood in the urine, urinating at night, pain on urination, or any sudden change in normal urinary habits.

These are the same symptoms that characterize BPH, with one important difference. If you have BPH, the symptoms develop gradually. With cancer, they may begin quite abruptly.

Prostate cancer also may produce a few symptoms not normally associated with BPH. Ejaculation may become painful. And since prostate cancer is the leading cause of bone metastases, which may cause back pain, unexplained back pain can also be a sign. The pain is usually in the spine, but it may also be in the bony pelvis, the lower back, the hips, or the bones of the upper legs.

Part of the problem in diagnosing prostate cancer is that the lack of early symptoms makes it hard to detect before it has spread. Another problem, according to the medical establishment, is that men don't show up dutifully for their annual digital rectal exams.

Even if they did, it might not be worth the trip. This is because the results of early-detection programs have been so disappointing, in terms of finding curable tumors, that some leading members of the medical community have concluded that mass screenings may not be worthwhile. In a comprehensive review in *Ca—A Cancer Journal for Clinicians*, published by the ACS, three researchers took a hard look at some of the statistics to date and concluded that there is "no clear evidence to suggest decreased mortality from any diagnostic test." (An exception may be the PSA test, discussed below.) Although there's an ongoing effort to refine the screening methods for prostate cancer, the tests—as well as the treatment—are all highly problematic.

Diagnosing Prostate Cancer

Let's discuss the tests one at a time: the rectal exam, the prostate-specific antigen (PSA) test, and **transrectal ultrasonography.**

RECTAL EXAMS

The historical view has been that rectal exams are a highly reliable means of catching most prostate cancers before they spread.

Unfortunately, there's a growing body of evidence to the contrary. Studies have shown that most patients have advanced disease by the time they're diagnosed by rectal exam. An analysis of the medical records of a large health maintenance organization in California, published in *Lancet* in 1991, concluded that "screening by routine digital rectal examination appears to have little if any effect in preventing metastatic prostatic cancer."

Another clinical study was even more devastating to the historical view. In this study, an annual rectal exam detected prostate cancer in 56 men—38 men in the first exam, 18 men the following year. Six years later six of the men who were diagnosed during the second rectal exam had died of prostate cancer. That works out to an exceedingly high mortality rate of 33 percent—compared with only 8 percent of the men whose cancer was detected during the initial exam.

The study suggested this might be because tumors that are small and confined to the prostate may be hard to detect by rectal exam. Another major reason is that many of the cancers start on the far side of the prostate, opposite the rectum, so they cannot be felt. The authors of the clinical study theorize that the tumors found in the second group were more aggressive and grew faster—hence the higher mortality rate.

The researchers suggested that if the rectal exam were performed more frequently than once a year, more of this aggressive cancer might be detected. However, given the high dropout rate in their own study, in which the exam was free, it's doubtful that stepping up the recommended number of digital exams would be very effective. An alternative, the researchers say, is that a more sensitive test may be required to detect these tumors when they're still curable. Such a test has not yet been developed.

Not all research, however, has had such uninspiring results. In an August 1998 study in *Urology,* researchers from the Mayo Clinic in Rochester, Minnesota, reported that DREs *can* save lives. They looked at the records of 173 men who died of prostate cancer and compared them with those of 350 peers who were still living. The men who died of the cancer were half as likely to have had regular DREs in the 10 years before they were diagnosed than were the men who were still living. According to the researchers, that suggests that screening may have prevented 50 to 70 percent of deaths that might have occurred from prostate cancer.

PROSTATE-SPECIFIC ANTIGEN (PSA) TEST

Prostate-specific antigen is a glycoprotein enzyme produced almost exclusively by the prostate and detectable in all men who have prostates and normal levels of testosterone. The level of the enzyme rises in men with prostate cancer. Studies have found that, gram for gram, the average prostate cancer produces at least 10 times the amount of PSA produced by normal prostatic tissue.

> ## At a Glance:
> ## Digital Rectal Exam Recommendations
>
> | Organization | Recommendation |
> |---|---|
> | American Cancer Society | A DRE should be done annually beginning at age 50 to men with a life expectancy of at least 10 years. Younger men at high risk may begin annual testing at an earlier age. |
> | National Cancer Institute | No recommendation can be made based on currently available evidence. |
> | U.S. Preventive Services Task Force | Annual DREs are not recommended. |

PSA levels, taken from blood samples, are stated in terms of nanograms, or billionths of a gram, per milliliter. A normal PSA level would be less than 4 ng/ml. A PSA level between 4 and 10 ng/ml is in the "gray area" that may indicate a local tumor. A level above 10 points strongly to cancer.

The PSA test is generally better at detecting prostate cancer than a rectal exam. In one major study involving 150,000 men, PSA was twice as accurate as the rectal exam in finding cancer. PSA accurately predicted cancer 40 percent of the time, whereas a positive rectal exam was correct only 20 percent of the time.

In fact, the PSA test might be able to indicate cancer before there's a palpable lump in the prostate. There's some indication that PSA levels start to rise, within the normal range, as many as 10 years before a tumor is diagnosed. A study at Johns Hopkins University, using stored serum, found a connection between small annual increases in PSA levels and a subsequent diagnosis of prostate cancer. While PSA levels tend to rise as men age, the rate of change was significantly greater in men who would eventually be diagnosed with prostate cancer.

The PSA test is a sensitive diagnostic tool. However, it's so sensitive, as we indicated in the previous section, that it's highly controversial. There are two major problems with the test.

First, the PSA test may give the wrong answer. PSA test results are often false negatives—that is, they're normal even if cancer is present. In studies, between 20 and 40 percent of men with localized prostatic cancers had normal PSA levels. False-positive results, or high levels of PSA when there's no cancer, are also common. Only one in three men with elevated PSA levels who undergo biopsies is found to have cancer.

A number of extraneous factors can result in false positives. If you have prostatitis, for example, your PSA level rises temporarily. A major trauma or injury to your prostate, such as an operation or biopsy, can increase your PSA level fiftyfold and keep it there for two weeks. Ejaculation also raises PSA levels for about two days. And although research indicates that a rectal exam has only a negligible effect on PSA levels, you may want to have blood drawn for a PSA before undergoing a DRE just to be on the safe side. Some feel the DRE may "squeeze" the prostate and release more of the antigen.

But the main reasons for false positives are age—which, as we noted earlier, causes elevated PSA levels—and the growth of benign prostatic tissue. An enlarged prostate produces more prostate-specific antigen. And since BPH is so common in the same age group that's at risk for prostate cancer, many in the medical community consider the PSA test unreliable for diagnosing prostate cancer.

To make the PSA test more reliable, researchers have been looking at different ways to evaluate and interpret the data. Some believe that calculating PSA density (the PSA concentration, divided by prostate volume as determined by ultrasound) may get around the problems caused by enlarged prostates. But one leading researcher, William Catalona, M.D., chief of urology at the Washington University School of Medicine, in St. Louis, argues that it would raise the cutoff point, making it likely that more cancers would be missed.

And to resolve the problem surrounding PSA levels and age, age-adjusted PSA reference ranges have been created. These ranges allow for higher PSA levels in older men, with a lower cutoff point for younger men. Age-specific reference ranges have also been designed for African-American men. (See tables.)

Age-Adjusted PSA Levels

Age	Acceptable PSA Level
40–49	2.5 ng/ml
50–59	3.5 ng/ml
60–69	4.5 ng/ml
70–79	6.5 ng/ml

Age-Adjusted PSA Levels for African-American Men

Age	Acceptable PSA Level
40–49	2.0 ng/ml
50–59	4.0 ng/ml
60–69	4.5 ng/ml
70–79	5.5 ng/ml

Other researchers maintain that the rate of change, or velocity, in PSA levels is a better predictor. According to those guidelines, an increase of more than 0.75 ng/ml per year may be indicative of cancer.

A diagnostic blood test, approved by the Food and Drug Administration in March 1998, is based on the finding that PSA exists in the blood in two forms: by itself in a free state or bound to other compounds in a complex state. Research indicates that a man with a higher percentage of free-state PSA is more likely to have benign prostatic hyperplasia than prostate cancer; in other words, the lower the percentage, the greater the risk of cancer. The free-state test comes in handy after a traditional PSA test comes back with high levels. If the test indicates a low percentage of free-state PSA, a biopsy to confirm or rule out cancer is recommended (we talk about biopsy later in this chapter). But a high percentage of free-state PSA indicates that BPH may be causing the elevated PSA levels.

A study headed by Catalona that was published in the May 20, 1998, *Journal of the American Medical Association* looked at 773 men with PSA levels between 4 and 10 ng/ml. By using a cutoff of 25 percent or less of free-state PSA for patients with PSA levels between 4 and 10 ng/ml, researchers were able to detect 95 percent of cancers while avoiding 20 percent of unnecessary biopsies. In addition, the cancers that were associated with a percentage of more than 25 percent were generally smaller and less advanced.

The other major problem with the PSA test is that it may tell you more than you need to know. No evidence to date shows that screening with a PSA test improves the health or extends the life of a man with prostate cancer. A critical issue is whether an early finding of cancer increases a man's life span or just his anxiety level. For older men with prostate cancer, many doctors believe, ignorance may be bliss. "The PSA test may identify many men with small, slow-growing cancers who will then want to be cured with treatments that may be more destructive than the tumors themselves," says Barry Kramer, M.D., associate director for the National Cancer Institute's Early Detection and Community Oncology Program.

Other doctors argue, however, that men should be informed about the PSA test and then decide what they want to do. Not every older man who learns he has prostate cancer will elect treatment.

The ability of the PSA test to prevent the spread of cancer is also up in the air. We quoted experts earlier who said diagnostic testing has not been proved to save lives. However, a long-term study presented by Canadian researchers at the May 1998 meeting of the American Society of Clinical Oncology reported that PSA testing can reduce the death rate due to prostate cancer by 69 percent. Unfortunately, the controversy isn't settled yet. Most researchers are not convinced that the study is accurate, citing problems with how the research was conducted.

Recommendations on the timing of routine PSA screening vary. The American Cancer Society, while conceding there are "recognized problems" with using PSA as a screening technique, recommends that all men age 50 and over have a PSA test each year along with their rectal exam. Men in the high-risk groups we mentioned earlier—for example, African American men and men whose fathers or brothers have had prostate cancer—should start annual screenings between ages 40 and 45. The ACS also stresses that men be given information on the potential risks (inaccurate results, overzealous treatment, and the like) and benefits (early detection of cancer) of screening. The American Urological Association offers similar recommendations.

But in its 1995 Guide to Clinical Preventive Services, the U.S. Preventive Services Task Force was highly critical of routine screening with PSA. "There is currently insufficient evidence to determine the need and optimal interval for repeat screening or whether PSA thresholds must be adjusted for density, velocity or age," the researchers concluded.

If screening is to be performed, the Task Force prefers screening with the rectal exam and PSA, but not ultrasound (which we discuss next), and limiting screening to men with a life expectancy greater than 10 years—that is, men under the age of 70. The Task Force's recommendation against screening is in line with recommendations in Great Britain, Canada, and New Zealand.

To further complicate matters, experts have recently presented evidence suggesting that routine PSA testing may take place every two years instead of every year, with no greater risk from cancer. One study, led by H. Ballentine Carter, M.D., of the Johns Hopkins University School of Medicine in Baltimore, found that symptom-free men ages 50 to 70 have a small chance of developing an incurable cancer during that additional year.

> ### At a Glance:
> ### Prostate-Specific Antigen Test Recommendations
>
> | Organization | Recommendation |
> |---|---|
> | American Cancer Society American Urological Association | A PSA test should be given annually beginning at age 50 to men with a life expectancy of at least 10 years. Younger men at high risk may begin annual testing at an earlier age. |
> | National Cancer Institute | No recommendation can be made based on currently available evidence. |
> | U.S. Preventive Services Task Force | Annual PSA tests are not recommended. |

At any rate, the choice is yours. Hundreds of medical centers, with underwriting from drug companies, have leapt onto the PSA bandwagon and are offering free PSA tests to screen for prostate cancer.

TRANSRECTAL ULTRASOUND

Ultrasound uses sound waves to create an image of a part of the body. In transrectal ultrasound (sometimes abbreviated as

> ## Beyond PSA?
>
> Researchers have identified a new substance that, like PSA, could help detect early cases of prostate cancer. The Physicians' Health Study from the Harvard University School of Public Health, published in the January 23, 1998 issue of *Science*, reported that men with high levels of the hormone insulin-like growth factor-1, called IGF-1, were more than four times as likely to develop prostate cancer as men with low levels of the substance.
>
> If the study's findings are confirmed, a screening test could be developed to check men for high levels of IGF-1, which could point to prostate cancer. Experts believe that IGF-1, which is produced by the liver, plays a part in the growth of prostate cancer.

TRUS), the ultrasound is sent out by a probe inserted into the rectum. The waves bounce off the prostate, and a computer uses the echoes to create a picture called a **sonogram.** Most prostate cancers appear less dense than the surrounding tissue.

Unfortunately, transrectal ultrasound is not very sensitive and has not been proved to be reliable. There are not much data on the role of ultrasound alone in detecting prostate cancer. And what data exist aren't terribly encouraging.

Preliminary results of the American Cancer Society National Prostate Cancer Detection Project, a study evaluating the use of all three screening methods in nearly 3,000 men, indicate that ultrasound is sensitive to a fault in detecting cancer. While ultrasound detected more tumors than rectal exams did in the study, it also yielded an appalling number of false positives (often in cases of BPH) and missed about one-quarter of the cancers. It also picked up a large number of tumors classified as premalignant that could probably be safely ignored for years, possibly forever.

Traditional ultrasound (performed through the abdomen rather than the rectum) is not used for a number of reasons. Some tumors simply don't show up well on ultrasound. Conversely, many areas that look like tumors are merely tissue that's inflamed.

Unlike a PSA level, a sonogram's meaning is in the eye of the beholder. When Fred Lee, M.D., director of the Prostate Center at Crittenton Hospital, in Rochester, Michigan, conducted his own studies of ultrasound as a means of detecting prostate cancer, his results were significantly more impressive than other researchers'. Lee, a veteran radiologist, complains that many urologists have acquired ultrasound equipment and are using it as a diagnostic tool but don't know how to read the sonogram.

Despite its drawbacks as an initial diagnostic method, ultrasound is valuable for directing a prostate biopsy. Using ultrasound, practitioners can see to guide and place biopsy needles to accurately sample suspicious tissue.

COMBINING THE TESTS

A combination of a rectal exam, PSA test, and transrectal ultrasound may be used to help diagnose prostate cancer with more success than from any one test. Studies indicate that the whole is greater than the sum of the parts—that is, that each test can detect tumors the other two may overlook and eliminate a number of the false-positive results or at least add more information to the diagnosis. In a preliminary report, researchers on the ACS National Prostate Cancer Detection Project conclude that "it may be possible to increase the early detection of prostate cancer substantially" through a combination of rectal exam, ultrasound, and PSA.

However, there's still no ironclad proof that, if you underwent all three tests every year, you'd increase your odds of surviving prostate cancer.

No one is sure what might be the most effective combination of tests. One study, in which some 1,700 men were tested, recommended the combination of PSA and rectal exam and, in patients with abnormal findings, ultrasound. But even that study's authors cautioned that their results hadn't established that such testing would improve survival rates.

In 1993, the NCI launched a 16-year clinical trial in which 37,000 men, ages 60 to 74, are being screened with rectal exams and PSA tests for prostate cancer. Positive results for either screen will lead to further diagnostic tests, including

The Search for the Prostate Cancer Gene

Experts around the world are currently in a race to discover the whereabouts of a gene (or several genes) that is thought to contribute to the development of hereditary prostate cancer. The location of one gene, known as HPC1, is already roughly known, and researchers predict they will uncover a precise chromosomal address sometime in the near future.

Pinpointing the gene would be important for several reasons. If it is located, it might become possible to screen men for the gene, identifying those at high risk for prostate cancer. Already such a test is available to screen women for the breast cancer genes known as BRCA1 and BRCA2.

Identifying the gene might also be useful in determining the course of the cancer, such as whether it is aggressive or slow growing—in fact, men with a family history of the disease tend to have more aggressive cancers, and they often fare worse after surgery. Genetic information could be used to tailor a treatment plan to the affected man's needs. In addition, understanding the gene and where it is located may help researchers discover more about why and how prostate cancer develops and, therefore, how to treat it. It might even be possible to develop a genetic therapy to combat the disease.

transrectal ultrasound. But any definitive answers to the questions about screening, including at what age it should take place and how frequently, are years away.

Determining Cancer's Spread

If a rectal exam, PSA test, or transrectal ultrasound is positive for cancer, the next step is to determine its stage. Diagnostic methods are important not only in determining whether cancer is present but also in determining its size, its rate of growth, and how far it has spread from its original location. All these factors come into play when you must decide among your treatment options.

When cancer is diagnosed, each tumor is classified, using the methods to be described shortly, as being in a specific stage based on its size, extent, location, and microscopic appearance. This process is called **staging.** Over time the tumor may progress through a series of stages. Many prostate cancers never spread; they remain completely localized within the prostatic capsule. If and when a tumor does metastasize, it moves initially to the neighboring organs. Eventually, it may also travel to the bone, lungs, chest, and even brain.

STAGES OF PROSTATE CANCER

There are several systems for grading prostate cancer, all based on what the tumor looks like and how it behaves. Until recently the most common system used four stages of prostate cancer: A, B, C, and D. Now, however, prostate cancer is staged according to the Tumor, Nodes, Metastases (TNM) System, using the abbreviations T1, T2, T3, T4, N, and M.

Stage T1 (previously stage A) is the earliest-stage tumor. This stage cancer is found incidentally, in tissue that's removed from enlarged prostates. It's too early to turn up on a rectal exam or any other screening test. It's a peculiar tumor; in some men it can be latent for decades, while in others it can advance so aggressively that it kills within a year or two. Usually, but not always, it's confined to the prostate.

Stage T2 (previously stage B) cancer is typically found during a routine rectal exam, when the doctor feels a hard or firm area of the prostate. The man himself is probably unaware there's a problem, because the cancer at this stage is contained within the prostate and not causing any symptoms.

Stage T3 and T4 (previously stage C) cancers have grown beyond the prostate. In stage T3, the cancer affects the prostatic capsule or seminal vesicles. T4 describes a cancer that has invaded adjacent structures other than the seminal vesicles—for example, the bladder neck or rectum.

Cancer that has spread to the pelvic **lymph nodes** is categorized as N (previously stage D1). If the cancer has spread, or metastasized, far from the prostate—for example, to the lungs, the bones, or the liver—it's stage M (previously stage D2).

The ACS estimates that 58 percent of prostate cancers are diagnosed at a local stage—T1 or T2. Some 18 percent of cancers aren't caught until they've reached stage T3 or T4. An estimated 11 percent of prostate cancers aren't detected until they've metastasized (stages N or M).

The likelihood of a cure for prostate cancer depends on what stage it has reached. It also depends on your definition of the word *cure*.

The ACS reports that the five-year survival rate with treatment is 100 percent for men whose tumors are still confined to the prostate when they're diagnosed. If the cancer has escaped the prostatic capsule, the survival rate over the next five years falls to about 94 percent. And if it has spread to the lymph nodes or bone or through the bloodstream to other organs, such as the liver or bladder, the five-year survival rate drops to 31 percent.

Because of the advanced age of most men diagnosed with prostate cancer, slowing the cancer's inexorable progress is a significant aspect of treatment for many men—as significant as destroying it when it's still vulnerable. In Chapter 6, we discuss the various treatments for prostate cancer, including the nontreatment option.

BIOPSY AND OTHER TESTS FOR STAGING

Most often cancer is confirmed and staged using a procedure called a biopsy. In a biopsy the doctor inserts a needle through the rectum, or sometimes the perineum, and into the prostate to remove a core of tissue. The procedure can be done in a doctor's office with minimal discomfort, and no anesthesia is required. Often a transrectal ultrasound is used during the procedure to create an image of the area and help guide the needle. Collected tissue is then examined under a microscope for cancer cells. Microscopic examination is the only way to make a definitive diagnosis. To determine the extent of the cancer, the doctor may do multiple biopsies to sample a wide area of prostate tissue.

Two recent inventions have made biopsy a relatively painless procedure that can be done without anesthesia. One is a spring-loaded biopsy "gun," which is guided by ultrasound through the rectum to suspicious areas of the prostate. The gun works so fast and uses such a fine needle that it's barely perceptible.

The other form of biopsy is a skinny-needle **aspiration**-type biopsy, in which cells are literally aspirated, or sucked, out of the gland through a very thin needle inserted through the rectum.

Biopsy is relatively safe, with one significant risk: Rectal bacteria can easily enter the prostate. Because of this risk, you are given antibiotics before the procedure to help ward off infection. Even so, you may get a persistent low-grade prostatitis that, as we discuss earlier in this chapter, can be hard to shake. (Men who already have prostatitis should not have a biopsy, according to Stephen N. Rous, the urologist-author of *The Prostate Book.*) An infection can also increase your PSA level, which makes it difficult to detect cancer in subsequent tests until the infection is finally cleared up.

A biopsy is appropriate for men whose rectal exams disclose irregularities or lumps; men whose PSAs are above 10 ng/ml; and men with telltale symptoms, such as sudden—rather than gradual—trouble urinating, bone pain, or suspicious x-rays or **bone scans.**

If you have medium-range PSA results, however, the need for a biopsy is less clear. Increasingly, doctors are automatically ordering biopsies and ultrasounds for men whose PSA levels are between 4 and 10 ng/ml, which some experts think is an overreaction. Expert radiologist Fred Lee, M.D., for example, believes too many biopsies are being done by urologists who don't know how to read ultrasounds. He advises, "Don't let anyone biopsy you just because your PSA is elevated." He urges men to get an ultrasound that's expertly read and that also measures the size of the prostate.

Another option is to have the specialized PSA test called the free-state PSA test, which is mentioned earlier in the chapter. By determining the percentage of free-PSA in the body, the test can help indicate whether a biopsy is necessary.

If the biopsy is positive for prostate cancer, the next task is to determine the stage, or extent, of the cancer. Is it contained in the prostatic capsule? Has it spread to the lymph nodes? Is it in the bones? Staging, or determining how far the cancer has advanced, is a critical part of the diagnosis because it determines treatment.

Historically, rectal exams were used for staging, but given their dismal record on diagnosis, you won't be surprised to hear that they weren't very accurate. Now there are several blood tests and imaging techniques that are far more effective. These tests look for signs of the cancer and then try to determine its location and how far it has spread.

The main blood test is that mixed blessing, the PSA. While it's controversial as a diagnostic technique, it gets more respect as a staging tool. Researchers have found that it's extremely accurate at predicting whether the cancer has reached its final stage: metastasis to bone.

A study at the Mayo Clinic of more than 850 men with newly diagnosed, untreated prostate cancer found that, of 561 men with PSA levels of 10 ng/ml or less and no bone pain, only three had abnormal results on bone scans. Of the 467 men whose PSA level was 8 or less, none had abnormal bone scans. For practical purposes, concluded Joseph Oesterling, M.D., the principal author, men with no bone pain and a PSA level below 10 can skip the scan.

If your biopsy is positive, your blood, urine, or prostatic secretions will be checked for prostatic acid phosphatase (PAP) levels. PAP is generally elevated (greater than 1 unit per liter, or U/L) in men with spreading prostate cancer. A high PAP level, however, doesn't necessarily mean metastatic prostate cancer. There are a number of other conditions that can raise the level: BPH, prostatitis, Paget's disease (a bone disorder), pneumonia, and hepatitis. Atromid-S, a drug taken to lower cholesterol levels in the blood, can have the same effect.

Even a rectal exam and prostatic massage, which we described earlier, can raise PAP levels. This is because the enzymes that make PAP can be produced by other body tissues, including the rectum. So when that area gets manipulated during a rectal exam, it may release these enzymes into general circulation and temporarily raise PAP levels. However, since rectal exams are no longer commonly used for staging, you probably won't have one around the same time as a PAP analysis.

There are a few other tests used in staging cancer. You probably will already have had a transrectal ultrasound, as part of either the diagnostic process or the biopsy. But if you haven't, then your doctor most likely will order one after a positive biopsy. He may also order one or two other imaging procedures.

One such procedure is a **computerized tomography (CT or CAT) scan,** a series of detailed pictures that are created by a computer linked to an x-ray machine. The scan can show whether the lymph nodes are swollen, which might mean the cancer has spread there. The other procedure, **magnetic**

resonance imaging (MRI), links a computer to a powerful magnet, instead of x-rays, to produce pictures of the prostate and nearby lymph nodes that may reveal abnormalities. And, of course, there's the bone scan.

A bone scan shows whether cancer has spread to the bone. When cancer spreads from prostate to bone, it attacks and partially destroys the bone. The body tries to repair the damage by laying down new bone in the damaged area. A bone scan can reveal that information months before a standard x-ray shows anything.

In a bone scan, a radioactive substance is injected into a vein in your arm and moves from the blood to the bone. If there are bones under repair because they've been damaged, they absorb the isotope. A counting machine similar to a Geiger counter scans the entire body and tallies the amount of isotope that's taken up by each bone. Each of these counts shows up as a dot on a screen or a monitor. A lot of counts or dots indicates that cancer has spread to that bone.

The bone scan is accurate, with one proviso: It isn't designed to show cancer, only bone repair. So a high count can also signal bone fractures or even arthritis. However, if you already have a positive biopsy, a high radioactive count is a pretty strong indication that the cancer has spread. And an x-ray can then show whether the bone looks normal or damaged—as it would be if you had arthritis, for example.

Staging may also involve surgery. The only way to tell for sure if the lymph nodes have cancer is to biopsy them. If all the other tests put your cancer in a gray zone, your doctor may want to perform a pelvic **lymphadenectomy,** a biopsy of the lymph nodes surrounding the prostatic area. This is a surgical procedure in which the abdomen is opened and suspicious tissue is removed. It may be analyzed while you're still on the operating table. Sometimes this is done right before a **radical prostatectomy,** the complete removal of the prostate gland, an operation we discuss in Chapter 6.

There are two alternatives to the open lymphadenectomy that you may find more acceptable. The least invasive—but also least accurate—is a **lymphangiogram,** in which dye is injected into the lymph system and travels to the pelvic area. At that point an x-ray can reveal cancer in the nodes. The other, newer approach involves **laparoscopy,** or the use of a small viewing tube to gain access to the interior of the abdomen. In a laparoscopic pelvic dissection, the doctor can remove and examine lymph nodes without the trauma of major surgery. The dissection can be understood, at the outset, to be purely a staging technique and not necessarily a commitment to a prostatectomy.

A new method of determining how far cancer has spread is with ProstaScint (capromab pendetide). This substance, developed by Cytogen Corporation, of Princeton, New Jersey, is injected intravenously and circulates throughout the body. On its trip through the system, it attaches to an antigen produced by prostate cancer cells. Using a scanner, physicians can then check the distribution of ProstaScint in the body to determine if the cancer is localized or if it has spread. It is intended to be used on men who have already been diagnosed with localized prostate cancer and are at high risk for the spread of the disease and on those who have already had prostate surgery but suspect a recurrence of cancer.

As you can see from this chapter, being diagnosed with prostate cancer is often difficult—both emotionally and from a medical point of view. Keep in mind, however, that diagnosis is only the beginning of your experience with prostate cancer. Once diagnosis has been done, treatment—outlined in the next chapter—is your main concern.

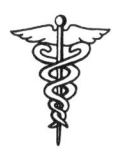

CHAPTER 6

Treatment of Prostate Cancer

THE MAIN TREATMENT OPTIONS FOR PROSTATE CANCER ARE SURGERY (usually a procedure called a radical prostatectomy), radiation therapy, hormonal therapy, and various combinations of all three. Still other treatments are more experimental. In this chapter, we discuss the full range of treatments.

Before we start, you should understand that not all treatments for prostate cancer are designed to cure the disease. Radical prostatectomies and radiation therapy are considered **curative** therapies, meaning that they may be capable of destroying the cancer altogether. Hormonal therapy is **palliative;** it can reduce the symptoms of the disease and slow its growth, but hormone therapy doesn't wipe it out.

If you're weighing different treatments for cancer, there's another term you should learn: **adjuvant.** Adjuvant treatment is any therapy that's offered after the most effective form of therapy has been tried.

Nontreatment is also an option—a very important one for many men. Because of their slow growth, some small, early-stage prostate cancers may not require treatment, especially if they're in men who are older or who have other serious illnesses. Other prostate cancers may be so far advanced that any treatment other than pain management may be useless and even cause suffering.

Furthermore, as we discuss later in this chapter, treatment is sometimes no more effective than watchful waiting. In summing up the "to treat or not to treat" dilemma, Willet F. Whitmore Jr., M.D., of Memorial Sloan-Kettering Cancer Center, in New York, has asked: "Is cure possible in those for whom it is necessary and is cure necessary in those for whom it is possible?"

We may get some answers from the Prostate Intervention Versus Observation Trial, launched by the National Cancer Institute. The trial seeks to compare the efficacy of radical prostatectomy (complete removal of the prostate gland) with watchful waiting in men with localized prostate cancer. However, results won't be available until the year 2010.

Once you've been diagnosed with prostate cancer, you will need to make decisions on what treatment is best for you. The kind of treatment you receive should depend on the stage of your disease, your age, and your overall condition. We discuss all these in this chapter.

Questions to Ask

In the following pages we talk about the different treatment options available for prostate cancer, their advantages, and their disadvantages. But a great deal of information should also come from straightforward, honest discussions with your practitioner. Ask your doctor the following questions in order to get the full scoop on your treatment options. Keep them in mind as you continue to read:

- Are there any additional tests that you recommend?
- Is it likely the cancer has spread beyond the prostate? If the cancer has spread, can it still be cured?
- What is the stage of my cancer?
- What is my prognosis based on the stage of my cancer and my treatment options?
- Do you recommend surgery for my condition? Why or why not?
- What type of surgery would be best, in your opinion?
- Are there any risks or side effects involved with the treatment you're recommending?
- Are there any other treatments that might be appropriate for me? Why or why not?

continues

> - What will happen if I don't have the treatment you're recommending?
> - What are the chances that I will face incontinence or erection problems? What about infertility?
> - Are any complementary or experimental treatments available that might help?
> - How long will it take for me to recover?
> - What are the chances that my cancer will come back after treatment?

You should keep in mind that there's great uncertainty, even within the medical profession, about which treatments are most appropriate for various forms of prostate cancer, especially for stages T1 and T2. In an editorial in the *Journal of the American Medical Association,* Whitmore wrote that the "optimal management of clinically localized prostatic cancer may be more a matter of opinion than a matter of fact." In other words, there are really no definitive guidelines.

If you find all this uncertainty disturbing, remember that it's generating a lot of work by researchers to find both causes and treatments, and their findings may ultimately benefit you. In the meantime, though, here is what we do know about surgery and other treatments for prostate cancer.

Surgery: Radical Prostatectomy

A radical prostatectomy is major surgery in which the entire prostate and the seminal vesicles (structures that contribute to sperm production) are removed. It's not to be confused with the very limited prostatectomies for benign prostatic hyperplasia (enlarged prostate) that we describe in the previous chapter, and it's not nearly as common—yet. One study found that, as a result of the increase in the rate of reported prostate cancer and improvements in the procedure, the number of radical prostatectomies for Medicare recipients rose nearly sixfold between 1984 and 1990.

A radical prostatectomy is a complicated operation that takes a few hours. After the prostate is removed, the urinary tract is essentially reconstructed. The bladder is brought down into the pelvis, and the bladder neck is stitched to the stump of the urethra at the point where the prostate gland was detached from it. This bridges the gap where the prostate had been and reestablishes the lower urinary tract.

There are two different approaches to a radical prostatectomy, similar to two approaches we describe in Chapter 4 for partial prostatectomies for BPH. One is retropubic, approaching the prostate from behind and under the pubic bone. The other is perineal, approaching the prostate through the perineum (the space between the scrotum and the anus).

Both approaches have their pros and cons. The retropubic prostatectomy has the advantage of allowing the surgeon to take out the lymph nodes for study by a pathologist before he continues—or, if the cancer has spread, doesn't continue—with the operation. That's not possible during a perineal prostatectomy, so a prostate cancer patient may need two separate procedures several days apart: an abdominal incision to check out his lymph nodes and a perineal incision to remove his prostate.

This may make it sound as if there's no reason to have the perineal approach. However, there are drawbacks to the retropubic approach too. The recovery is harder, because an abdominal incision is considerably more uncomfortable than a perineal incision. And with the retropubic approach, it's somewhat more difficult to expose and remove the prostate.

Recovery may be difficult after a radical prostatectomy. There's considerable pain immediately afterward. You'll have bladder spasms and, because your intestine isn't contracting normally at first, you'll have a tube draining your abdomen for a few days. A Foley catheter, which we described earlier, is inserted through your penis and into your bladder for about three weeks after the operation. When the catheter is removed, you may be somewhat incontinent for several weeks or even months.

WHO CAN HAVE A RADICAL PROSTATECTOMY?

Radical prostatectomies are best for men with cancers that meet two conditions. First, the cancer must be encapsulated within the prostate. Men with stages T1 and T2 cancer are the main candidates for radical prostatectomies.

If your lymph nodes are found to be cancerous while you're on the table for a radical prostatectomy, you'll probably be stitched up at once and sent on to a recovery room. When you come to, you and your doctor will have to discuss what other treatments, such as hormone therapy, you can try.

But we should note that increasingly doctors are proceeding with the prostatectomy anyway. One reason is that the surgery itself has become safer for patients, with less risk of complications and death. In addition, some experts believe a prostatectomy is beneficial even when the cancer has already spread.

There's disagreement on that point. The traditional view is that, when the cancer has metastasized, there's nothing to be gained—and a lot of unnecessary suffering to be undergone—from removing the prostate. However, some researchers believe that, since new deposits of cancer can come only from the original site, it may be useful to attack the cancer in the prostate.

Research done by the Mayo Clinic evaluated the impact of radical prostatectomy on advanced cancer patients who also had their testicles removed. (As we discuss later, testicle removal is one kind of hormonal therapy.)

The researchers reported a better survival rate for men who undergo combined therapies rather than hormonal therapy alone. At the end of five years, men who'd had both their prostates and their testicles removed had a 91 percent survival rate, compared with 66 percent for men who'd had only their testicles removed. At 10 years the rates were 78 percent and 39 percent, respectively.

The second condition for a radical prostatectomy is the unofficial age cutoff. The unofficial consensus (one echoed, in fact, in the prostate cancer treatment guidelines of the National Cancer Institute) among doctors seems to be that a man over the age of 70 shouldn't have the operation because it probably wouldn't give him many, if any, additional years and might even subtract from what he's got left.

To put it bluntly, treatment is determined by a man's age simply because an older man is more likely to die of something else—a stroke or heart disease, for example—before prostate cancer does him in. Maybe you don't like the idea that doctors are making actuarial calculations worthy of insurance companies. But the fact is that many would consider it harsh to subject a man to treatment for prostate cancer if the tumor isn't likely to be the cause of his death.

Another reason that's given sometimes is that prostatic cancer is more aggressive in younger men. However, research now indicates that prostate cancer doesn't grow any faster in young men than it does in senior citizens.

The practice of not treating men over a certain age may sound like age discrimination. However, research says, the trend away from prostatectomy in older patients is dictated partly by patients themselves and partly by concern over their ability to tolerate therapy. In other cases, the doctors may have arbitrarily chosen 70 as the cutoff. Whether or not that's fair is a question we'll leave to medical ethicists. But it's worth noting that more people are recognizing two concerns: that treatment may be ineffective or even counterproductive and that health care resources are limited.

This doesn't mean that if you're 70, you won't be able to get a prostatectomy or shouldn't have one. Doctors are aware that although the life expectancy from birth of an American man is around 73, once he reaches that age he can expect to live another 10 years. And more and more men are living to the age of 90 and beyond. In *The Prostate Book,* Stephen N. Rous, M.D., says that "when a patient is in excellent condition and he is a physiological age 65 even though a chronological 75, I think that exceptions should be made."

RISKS AND COMPLICATIONS

Age and the stage of cancer at diagnosis are important factors in choosing a treatment for prostate cancer. But you also need to consider the risks and problems that may come with the procedures you're considering. With radical prostatectomy, as with any major surgery, there are risks. Studies show that about 1 percent of patients die from the procedure, and that's when

Safety in the Hospital

While in the hospital, you are at risk of acquiring a condition you did not have when you went in—called iatrogenic disease (*iatrogenic* is from the Greek, meaning "doctor-caused" or "doctor-produced").

One form of iatrogenesis is nosocomial infection. Acquired during hospitalization, nosocomial infections are produced by microorganisms that dwell within hospitals. In other words, you don't have the infection when you check in; you get it while you are there. Not only do such infections jeopardize your recovery, but the cost of their treatment may increase your hospital bill. To help prevent infections:

- Try to make sure that all hospital personnel who come in contact with you have washed their hands. If you so desire, ask them to do so in your room, in your presence. You can greatly lower your chances of catching an infection—and paying for its treatment.

- If your roommate becomes infected or if you are concerned that what he has could possibly be transmitted to you via the air or through the use of a common bathroom, ask your doctor about your risks.

- If you are undergoing surgery or a procedure that requires the removal of hair, refuse to be shaven the night before surgery. One study indicates that among people shaved the day prior to their operations, the nosocomial infection rate was 5.6 percent. Chemical depilatories reduce the rate to just 0.6 percent. Using barber clippers to remove hair the morning of surgery yields a low infection rate too.

- Have nurses regularly check the drainage of urinary catheters to help you maintain cleanliness.

Another form of iatrogenesis is the medication error. Surveys have shown medication errors to be common in hospitals across the United States. Some $76.6 billion a year is spent on drug errors. Adverse drug events occur at rates ranging from 0.2 per 100 admissions to 10 per 100 admissions.

You can prevent dangerous medication errors while in the hospital by being alert about the medications you take. The following guidelines from the American Society of Hospital Pharmacists (ASHP) can be used to avoid medication errors during a hospital stay:

- Inform all your health-care providers (physicians, nurses, and pharmacists) of your known allergies, sensitivities, and current medications.

- Ask questions about any recommended procedures and treatments.

- Learn the names of all drug products that are prescribed and administered to you.

continues

> - Keep track of the medications. Record all drug therapy, including prescribed drugs, nonprescription drugs, home remedies, and special diets.
>
> - Be assertive if something seems incorrect or different from the norm. For example, if you receive a different pill from the one you were expecting (for example, a red pill instead of a green pill), ask why. Also ask if you have not been given medication you are expecting.
>
> - Take prescription medication as prescribed. If possible, bring your prescription medications to the hospital with you and make arrangements with your doctor and the nursing station to take them according to schedule. The hospital may request that you sign a release form.

it's performed at top-rated hospitals. There's also a slight risk of infection, **fistula,** or rectal injury and a higher risk—between 9 and 18 percent—of bladder stricture, or scarring.

Risks increase with age. A study led by Grace Lu-Yao, Ph.D., for the Prostate Patient Outcomes Research Team, reported in 1993 that, among men over age 75 who had radical prostatectomies, almost 2 percent died and nearly 8 percent suffered major cardiopulmonary complications within 30 days of surgery.

There's also the question of the risk of impotence. A decade or two ago virtually all prostatectomies resulted in impotence.

Surgeons didn't recognize that a pair of nerve bundles close to the prostate control erections, so they inadvertently stretched or tore the nerves during radical prostatectomies. Then, in 1982, Patrick Walsh, M.D., a urologist at the Johns Hopkins University School of Medicine, identified the cobweblike nerves and devised the nerve-sparing procedure that allows surgeons to remove the prostate while leaving the nerves intact.

Now, while most men take several months to two years to recover full potency, permanent impotence after nerve-sparing surgery is the exception rather than the rule. In fact, radical prostatectomies, when appropriate, are more likely to be recommended for men who are still potent and healthy than are other treatments, which have a higher rate of impotence.

Age has much to do with the risk of impotence. At a conference of the American Urological Association in early 1997, Walsh said that 90 percent of patients in their forties will remain potent after the nerve-sparing surgery. For men in their fifties, sixties, and seventies, the rates stand at 75 percent, 60 percent, and 25 percent, respectively, under optimal conditions and with a surgeon who has mastered the technique.

Not all studies regarding impotence have had such promising outcomes. A 1997 study from Harvard Medical School, in Boston, that compared nerve-sparing surgery to traditional prostatectomy found that most men, regardless of the procedure they underwent, were impotent a year later. Only 21 percent of

> ## New Device May Save Nerves
>
> Surgeons may now get some help in locating the delicate nerves that, if severed, could cause impotence in men undergoing radical prostatectomy.
>
> The CaverMap, a machine developed at Harvard University, detects nerves as a metal detector detects metal. The closer the surgeon's knife comes to the nerves, the faster the machine beeps, alerting the doctor to the presence of the microscopic structures. UroMed, the corporation that will manufacture the CaverMap device, reported that, in one study, 92 percent of men who underwent radical prostatectomy had regained potency a year after surgery. The previous rate of that same surgeon had been 30 percent before CaverMap.
>
> The device was approved by the Food and Drug Administration in late 1997 and is currently available.

19 men who had bilateral nerve-sparing prostatectomies and none of the 12 men who had unilateral nerve-sparing prostatectomies was still potent one year later. In addition, more men who had nerve-sparing surgery experienced incontinence compared with those who had the traditional procedure.

The researchers conducting the study do recommend nerve-sparing surgery but caution that the procedure may not be as effective at reducing impotency as some think. They also suggest that outcomes would have been better had the operations been performed by surgeons who performed more than one of the procedures a year, which was the average in the study.

As Barry E. Epstein, M.D., a radiation oncologist at Fox Chase Cancer Center, in Philadelphia, has noted tactfully, "There is as yet no evidence that the average urologist performs the anatomic [nerve-sparing] radical prostatectomy with outcomes comparable to those of the few centers of surgical expertise that publish results." In other words, if you're considering a nerve-sparing prostatectomy, find a surgeon with plenty of experience with the procedure.

You'll also want to find a surgeon with a light touch—and not just for the sake of your nerves. Researchers say gentle handling of the prostate during prostatectomy is important in preventing the release of cancer cells into the bloodstream, which may increase the risk of metastatic disease.

Because nerve-sparing prostatectomy makes an effort to preserve the nerves that control erections, there's been some concern that surgeons have been leaving behind cancerous cells. While that hasn't been proved, research has found that nerve-sparing prostatectomies left positive margins in 75 percent of men with stage T3 or T4 cancer. So some experts believe that nerve-sparing surgery should be reserved for younger men with tumors in the earlier stages.

Prostatectomy and Impotence

If you have the prostatectomy and do become impotent, all is not necessarily lost. Any man can regain the ability to have rigid erections, depending on his willingness to try mechanical solutions or other methods. There are several kinds of treatments, ranging from oral medicines and penile injections to vacuum devices and prostheses.

The recently approved drug sildenafil (better known as Viagra) is fast becoming the most widely used remedy for impotence. The drug works by blocking an enzyme that causes erections to fade. Early studies have shown the drug to be effective for about half the people who use it. Reported side effects include headache, backache, and indigestion.

Before sildenafil, most men treated impotence with self-injection. With this method, a man injects into his penis a couple of drops of a drug (papaverine, phentolamine, or prostaglandin E1—also called alprostadil or Caverject) that relaxes arterial muscles and allows blood to flow into the penis. A pellet form of alprostadil that is inserted into the urethra with a special applicator is also available.

Among other treatments for impotence is a vacuum device that puts negative pressure on the penis, making it bigger and longer. A tight rubber band is then applied to the base of the penis, holding the erection in place.

A penile prosthesis is a device that, when surgically implanted within the body, allows an impotent man to have erections for intercourse. There are three types of penile prostheses available: malleable rod; self-contained hydraulic; and inflatable, an elaborate device designed to mimic as closely as possible the process of an erection.

An inflatable prosthesis, in addition to the penile implant, involves a fluid-filled reservoir, which is implanted under the abdominal muscles, and a pump, placed in the scrotum. When the man wants an erection, he squeezes the pump, moving fluid from the reservoir to the cylinders. When he presses another site on the pump, the fluid leaves the cylinders and returns to the reservoir, and the penis relaxes.

Each treatment has its pros and cons. You're probably shuddering at the notion of sticking a needle into your penis, but it's reportedly not as bad as you think; you inject into the side, where there's spongy tissue with no nerve endings. Still, there are risks. Injections may lead to uncomfortable scarring. If you inject too much of the drug, the erection may last too long and kill penile tissue.

The vacuum device is simple and safe. It's often preferred by older men who don't insist on completely rigid erections. For a number of reasons, the prostheses have fallen out of favor recently. They require surgery, which is expensive and can lead to complications, and there's always a slight risk that the device may

continues

> malfunction. Some doctors prescribe them as a last resort for men who can't or won't use the other methods.
>
> You can obtain more information about treatment for impotence from one of the groups listed at the end of this book.

The risk of incontinence is now lower with the nerve-sparing approach to radical prostatectomies, thanks to several modifications. In the same study we cited earlier, Walsh reported that 92 percent of the patients had recovered complete urinary control and 6 percent had mild stress incontinence—a condition we describe in Chapter 4. The problem was more severe in another 2 percent, but no one was totally incontinent. More recent studies have not been as optimistic. A study published in the April 1996 *Journal of Urology* reported that 40 percent of men have daily incontinence after prostatectomy. Another study reported at the 1997 meeting of the Gerontological Society of America estimated the rate to be 63 percent.

One complication that isn't likely to bother most men with prostate cancer, but should be noted for the record, is that men are permanently sterile after radical prostatectomies. This is because removal of the entire prostate gland, including the prostatic urethra, eliminates any place that the sperm can be deposited. So as part of the operation, the vas deferens are tied off.

All Is Not Said and Done . . .

Keep in mind that radical prostatectomy does not guarantee that you will never need future treatment for prostate cancer. In some men, cancerous cells are left behind after the surgery; in others, the cancer may have spread beyond the prostate even before surgery. Further treatment usually comes in the form of radiation or hormonal therapy.

A 1996 study from Dartmouth, Harvard, the University of Connecticut, and the National Cancer Institute reports that 34 percent—about one-third—of men who had the procedure required treatment within the next five years. The study may overstate the retreatment rate, however, because it includes information on men treated before the advent of the PSA test, which diagnoses prostate cancer earlier, when it is less likely to have spread. Other experts report the rate to be more like 10 percent. Whatever the rate, however, researchers warn that men thinking about prostatectomy should factor in the possibility of retreatment.

If cancer has spread beyond the prostate or there's a chance cancerous cells were missed, radiation or hormonal therapy may be recommended after a radical prostatectomy to eradicate any remaining cells. If the surgery was for a cure, and the surgeon tells you he got the tumor out, you may not receive further treatment. It's not uncommon, however, for men with early-stage cancer to undergo radiation after a radical prostatectomy. Many studies have

continues

> shown that the combination reduces the rate of recurrence in the region where the prostate was, and there are indications that it improves the rate of survival.
>
> Hormonal therapy would be prescribed as adjuvant treatment—that is, it would be used if, despite the prostatectomy and/or radiation, the tumor spreads outside the prostatic capsule.

Cryosurgery

There's some interest in cryosurgery, the low-temperature technology we talk about in Chapter 4. In this procedure, probes filled with liquid nitrogen are inserted into the prostate via the urethra. They freeze and destroy the entire prostate, as well as the surrounding tissue and structures such as the seminal vesicles if they're also cancerous. The dead tissue is left in place and eventually reabsorbed by the body. The use of ultrasound and temperature-sensitive probes has helped refine the procedure.

So far, the success rate of cryosurgery has been promising, though the therapy is still too new to evaluate. In addition, patients recover quickly because the procedure does not require an incision and there is little blood loss.

Cryosurgery is helpful for men with early-stage tumors and those who can't undergo more conventional treatment because they're too ill or have already had surgery or radiation. One of cryosurgery's major advantages, compared with those two options, is that it can be performed more than once on patients who still have cancer after initial treatment. However, rates of impotence are quite high—hovering around 94 percent, says one 1997 study. For this reason, cryosurgery is usually recommended for patients older than 70.

If the therapy continues to produce good results, says Gary Onik, M.D., an interventional radiologist at Allegheny General Hospital, in Pittsburgh, where cryosurgery has been used effectively, "it will be the first-line treatment of choice." At this point, however, it's still considered experimental and may not always be covered by insurance.

Radiation Therapy

In treating prostate cancer, **radiation therapy**, or radiotherapy, uses high-energy rays to shrink tumors and stop cancer cells from growing. Like surgery, it's local therapy—that is, it affects only the cells in the treated area.

There are several kinds of radiation therapy. All are administered by a radiologist (a specialist in administering radiation and interpreting x-rays) or radiation oncologist (a subspecialist in radiology who deals specifically with radiation therapy and cancer), who plan and supervise the treatment. The more common is **external-beam radiotherapy,** in which a machine aims rays at the tumor and the pelvic area. Typically, a man receives this radiation by going to a hospital five days a week for six or seven weeks.

External-beam radiotherapy may produce side effects such as diarrhea, cramping, and intestinal ulcers, all of which typically clear up within weeks after treatment ends. It has also led, in various studies, to permanent impotence in 20 to 50 percent of the men who undergo treatment.

Radiation therapy usually causes fatigue, and the kinds of therapy used in prostate cancer are no exception. Unlike other forms of radiation, though, radiation for prostate cancer doesn't have nausea or burns among its side effects. With external-beam radiation, the skin over the target area may turn red or become dry. But because the radiation is aimed precisely, patients don't get the burns, hair loss, or nausea that often result when other parts of the body are irradiated. And there's no indication that it causes other tumors to develop.

A variation of external-beam radiation is proton therapy, in which a beam of high-energy proton particles is precisely aimed at the prostate gland. The beam delivers high doses of radiation to the cancerous areas while sparing normal tissue. This therapy is best used for localized cancers that have not spread throughout the body. Side effects are negligible and may include fatigue, nausea, and diarrhea.

Another kind of radiation therapy is delivered internally by radioactive material that's implanted as "seeds" or "pellets" in and around the prostate. Internal radiation therapy is also known as **brachytherapy** or **interstitial radiation therapy.**

There is a growing variety of implants. Some are left in place permanently, while others are removed after they've served their purpose. The kind of tumor determines the choice of implant. Some names you may hear are palladium-103 and iodine-125, two widely used permanent implants that emit low-energy radiation over a period of a couple of weeks or a couple of months, respectively; gold-198, which releases energy at an extremely high rate for a few days; and iridium-192, a high-energy temporary implant.

The seeds can be injected through needles with the help of ultrasound or by means of an open procedure (a surgery that involves an incision)—either suprapubic or retropubic. If the doctor uses needles, it's a quick procedure under a spinal anesthetic. As many as 100 rice-sized seeds may be implanted in an hour.

Walking around with radioactive isotopes sounds dangerous. Initially, however, you wouldn't be walking around a lot. With iridium-192, you'd probably be quarantined in a hospital room for at least two months, with special precautions to protect nursing staff. With lower-energy implants, you'd be sent home but told to remain somewhat isolated from other people to avoid exposing them to excess doses of radiation. For the first 17 days of palladium, for example, you must keep your distance from pregnant women and not let a young child sit in your lap for more than five minutes at a time.

How long you're sequestered depends on the half-life of the implant (the length of time that it's highly radioactive). Once the radioactivity wears off, however, you don't need to worry about exposing others. Men with permanent implants can have sexual intercourse with no risk to their partners.

Implants don't usually lead to impotence, but there are sometimes severe complications, such as perforated rectums, when the seeds are implanted. And they have been blamed for temporary urinary difficulties similar to those of BPH.

Choosing between the different forms of radiation and then making a further choice among the various implants is a highly complicated decision that ultimately must be left to the experts. It depends primarily on the kind of tumor that's being treated. Increasingly, implants are being used to treat large, bulky tumors, to ensure that the radiation is delivered primarily to the tumor rather than to normal tissue.

External radiotherapy and brachytherapy are often combined if the implants are temporary. One of the implants we've mentioned, iridium-192, has been combined with external-beam radiation in several studies. In one of the largest studies, at California's Long Beach Memorial Medical Center, researchers reported an excellent survival rate for men who had the combined therapies. Other experts caution, however, that more studies are needed to confirm that the combination is really superior to conventional external-beam radiation alone.

Some men may have reasons—aside from tumor type—to choose one radiation therapy over the other. Not everybody can use implants. It's out of the question for a man whose rectum has been removed, because the prostate probe has to be placed through the rectum. Men can't have implants if they have large prostates (and would need too many seeds) or have had prior prostate surgery and don't have enough tissue to hold the seeds.

The traditional view is that radiation therapy should be limited to men whose cancer is confined to the prostate and surrounding tissues. That's stages T1 and T2. Some doctors believe, however, that radiation is also effective when the cancer has spread to local lymph nodes. That's stage N. A study by researchers at the Medical College of Wisconsin reported that, when N patients received radiation, 61 percent were disease-free at 5 years, and 48 percent at 10 years.

Whether surgery or radiation is the better choice depends on several factors, including who's doing the procedure. Patients who receive radiation tend to have much the same outcome regardless of where they're treated, while—as we said earlier—a person undergoing nerve-sparing prostatectomy fares better in the hands of an expert surgeon.

Studies show that, for men with stages T1 and T2 cancer, external radiation, brachytherapy, and radical prostatectomy seem to produce the same outcome over a 15-year period. Studies also show that for more aggressive disease, brachytherapy may be more effective than radical prostatectomy, which works best when the cancer is in its earliest stages.

Brachytherapy is growing in popularity for another reason: cost. The radioactive implants cost an estimated 60 percent less than either radical prostatectomy or external radiation. Brachytherapy is estimated to cost $7,000 to $12,000, while prostatectomy runs $15,000 to $20,000. Experts think the savings may cause insurance companies to push for brachytherapy over other forms of treatment.

As with radical prostatectomy, there is no guarantee that radiation therapy will completely eradicate your cancer. Residual cancer is microscopic tumors found by biopsy several months after the treatment. This doesn't mean that the tumor has recurred but rather that cells were left behind when the prostate was removed. It's difficult to eradicate cancer completely. Residual cancer has been reported in 30 to 50 percent of men who had radical prostatectomies and in 60 to 90 percent of men who had radiation therapy.

Residual cancer is not necessarily fatal. While failure to "cure" can be fatal in other cancers, it's not at all clear how dangerous it is in the case of prostate cancer. Autopsy studies have shown that about one-third of men over the age of 50 have microscopic evidence of prostate cancer.

However, if the PSA level—that measure of tumor growth that we discuss in Chapter 5—is elevated or rising, there's a good chance both you and your doctor will want to make another attack on the cancer with an adjuvant therapy, such as hormonal therapy.

Hormonal Therapy

As we discuss in Chapter 5, prostate cancer depends on androgens, or male hormones, to grow. Hormonal therapy deprives the cancer cells of androgens. Unlike radical prostatectomy or radiation, it's systemic therapy, meaning that it can reach cancer cells throughout the body.

There are two forms of hormonal therapy, and sometimes they're administered together. One involves taking hormones that stop the testicles from producing testosterone, the principal androgen. The other involves surgery.

The surgical approach is a **bilateral orchiectomy,** a procedure in which both testes are removed, generally through a single incision in the scrotal bag. That eliminates the main source of male hormones. It's a very simple procedure that can be done under local anesthesia and, because the scrotum is surprisingly insensitive to pain, causes little postoperative discomfort. So that the scrotum appears intact, some men choose to have prostheses: soft plastic balls that resemble the testicles in size and consistency.

Though you might expect the other hormonal therapy to involve estrogen, it does not. Estrogen therapy isn't used much anymore, partly because it's been established that it increases a man's risk of heart problems, including the formation of blood clots. The therapy that's overtaken estrogen and, increasingly, orchiectomy, is **luteinizing hormone-releasing hormone (LHRH) analog.**

LHRH is a hormone that normally controls the production of sex hormones. LHRH analogs, which are made in the laboratory, are like LHRH but instead prevent the testicles from producing testosterone.

LHRH analogs are given by daily or monthly injection. One widely used LHRH analog is leuprolide (sold as Lupton by TAP Pharmaceuticals); another is goserelin (sold as Zoladex by Zeneca). A new formulation of Zoladex, also given subcutaneously, is absorbed over a three-month, as opposed to one-month, period.

When used in combination with radiation, LHRH analogs are thought to be helpful for those with locally advanced prostate cancer—a stage of cancer that often doesn't do well with other therapies. Studies show that goserelin combined with radiation therapy has a greater five-year survival rate (79 percent) than does radiation therapy alone (62 percent) in men whose cancer has begun to spread.

LHRH analogs do not work immediately. Strangely enough, when they're first taken, they lead to higher testosterone levels and tumor growth, or what's known as "flare." This actually worsens some symptoms, including pain. But after about a week, testosterone levels fall to near zero, about the level achieved when both testes are removed. Tumor growth slows down, and the patient's condition improves.

The adrenal glands still produce small amounts of male hormones while LHRH is being taken. Sometimes the patient is given pills that contain an **antiandrogen,** a drug that blocks the effect of any remaining male hormones. These antiandrogens include flutamide (brand name Eulexin, manufactured by Schering-Plough), bicalutamide (brand name Carodex, by Zeneca), and finasteride, which we describe in Chapter 4 as a treatment for BPH. The newest antiandrogen drug is nilutamide (Nilandron, by Hoechst Marion Roussel).

Somewhat of a controversy has developed over whether these two kinds of hormone drugs are really necessary. The Food and Drug Administration approved the combined therapy in 1989, after studies showed that men treated with both typically lived for 35 months after treatment rather than the average 28 months. However, other studies have found little or no benefit in using antiandrogens except to suppress the initial tumor flare during the first week or so after patients start the LHRH analog.

There are, of course, some side effects of hormonal therapy. Many men (perhaps you're among them!) expect the worst: a high soprano voice, enlarged breasts, loss of facial hair. Happily, those are no longer side effects. Men may get hot flashes with both LHRH analog and orchiectomy. These can be extremely bothersome, but to an extent they can be treated with medication. Sometimes incontinence is a complication.

Men who receive estrogen or an antiandrogen may have nausea, vomiting, or tender and swollen breasts. These side effects can also be treated.

Hormonal therapy results in impotence far more often than nerve-sparing prostatectomies do. Both types of hormonal therapies are considered castration: One is surgical; the other is medical. Most men are impotent after hormonal therapy, and even those who aren't may lose sexual desire.

The psychological effects of an orchiectomy can be traumatic. Most men dread and fear the prospect of an orchiectomy, according to many veteran urologists. To many men, even elderly men who haven't had sexual relations for years, an orchiectomy is nothing less than emasculation. So is therapy with hormones, of course—but in theory, at least, that's reversible. An orchiectomy is not.

Another drawback to hormone therapy is that taking hormones is extremely expensive. A monthly shot of an LHRH analog costs more than $300. Throw in an antiandrogen, and you're looking at upwards of $500 a month. A bilateral orchiectomy, on the other hand, costs between $2,000 and $3,000, including surgeon's fees and associated hospital costs. That's a range for the country; obviously, you may pay more in some regions than in others.

If your health insurance doesn't cover the cost or if you don't have health insurance, you may be eligible to receive the drugs you need through an "indigent needs" program offered by pharmaceutical companies to those who meet specific low-income requirements. Usually, you must apply through your personal physician, who should then contact a local pharmaceutical sales representative for the necessary application forms and instructions. For more information, ask your physician.

The traditional candidates for hormone therapy are men whose cancer has spread outside the prostatic capsule to the lymph nodes, other tissues or organs, or to bone. Doctors may also recommend it to men with stage C cancer who can't have surgery or radiation. They might receive hormonal therapy, for example, if they're having trouble urinating because their tumors are compressing their urethras.

Some researchers theorize that because prostate cancer evidently requires the presence of androgens for growth, hormonal therapy should be used when the cancer is still in its early stages. However, there aren't any studies that support early use.

Orchiectomy and injections are equally effective in controlling prostate cancer, say clinical studies, so the decision between treatments comes down partly to economics, partly to personal preference. One study produced the unsurprising finding that, faced with a choice between orchiectomy and injections, a large majority of men chose injections.

Drug Therapy

Until recently, there were no drugs that acted directly on a prostate tumor. But now researchers are getting some interesting results with an experimental drug called suramin, which was first used decades ago against a tropical parasite.

In clinical trials, the National Cancer Institute has given suramin to 38 men whose prostate cancers had resisted hormonal treatment and had begun to spread to other tissues. NCI found that men treated with the drug had an 85 percent probability of living at least one year, compared with a 20 percent probability for men who didn't receive suramin.

Another study, by researchers at the University of Maryland, reports that suramin appeared to shrink the prostate gland—and thus, presumably, the tumor—in about three-quarters of 33 men with metastatic prostate cancer.

Less promising results stemmed from a study from the Jonsson Comprehensive Cancer Center at the University of California at Los Angeles. Researchers there found suramin to be effective for only 25 to 30 percent of men with metastatic prostate cancer. Further research is underway to find out why the studies differed so greatly in their results.

Suramin can have some powerful side effects. Among other things, it can damage the adrenal glands, which are on top of the kidneys and help regulate blood pressure by controlling water retention. In the Maryland drug trials, although researchers used a new computer-aided method of tailoring dosages to individual patients, the side effects were so severe that treatment had to be limited in 28 of the 37 patients. (The other four patients had different types of advanced cancers.)

Chemotherapy, which involves the use of different chemicals or drugs to kill cancer cells, hasn't proved too successful against prostate cancer. Sometimes it's administered to patients who have responded poorly to hormone therapy, as a means of controlling pain. To date, there's no evidence that it prolongs survival.

The drawbacks of chemotherapy depend in part on which drugs are used. In general, people who receive chemotherapy may find that they're more susceptible to infection. Other side effects can include loss of appetite, nausea, vomiting, or mouth sores. Patients may also have less energy and may lose their hair.

Other Therapies

A few therapies have not yet been touched upon. Biological therapies, which include biological response modifiers (BRM) and immunotherapy, are different from chemotherapy because they try to increase your own body's ability to fight the cancer.

Probably the best-known BRM therapy involves interferons, chemicals the body makes as a normal response to viral or other infections. A person with cancer may be given much larger amounts of interferon, made in biotechnology laboratories, to boost, direct, or restore his body's natural defenses against the tumor.

Immunotherapy uses antibodies that recognize and attach themselves to the tumor and kill cancer cells. To increase the effectiveness of this approach, antibodies may be linked to radioactive compounds or to chemotherapy drugs. Biological therapies are still in the experimental stage, and their roles in treating prostate cancer are unknown.

Other experimental therapies include differentiation therapy (using chemicals to stop cell reproduction and lower cell resistance to treatment) and the use of endothelin-1 agonists (to neutralize the pain-causing chemical endothelin-1). Researchers have also begun testing tumor vaccines, which consist of genetically modified genetic cells designed to stimulate the body's immune system to attack prostate cancer cells. Again, the effectiveness of these treatments is unknown. As far as side effects go, biological therapies tend to cause flulike symptoms, such as chills, fever, muscle aches, weakness, loss of appetite, nausea, vomiting, or diarrhea.

Alternative therapies can be enlisted in the fight against prostate cancer. Many of the alternative techniques that have been used against other cancers, such as biofeedback and visualization—in which you use your mind to try to control the spread of, or even to shrink, the tumor—obviously can be tried with prostate cancer. These can be learned from some psychotherapists.

Prostate Cancer Vaccines

Most people think of vaccines as protection against diseases such as measles, mumps, and polio. But researchers are giving the word *vaccine* a whole new meaning as they look for ways to jump-start men's immune systems in the fight against advanced prostate cancer.

The prostate vaccine is not a vaccine in the true sense. It's often referred to as such because it boosts a cancer patient's immune response against the disease and because it is administered in a series of injections.

Here's how it works. One of the problems associated with treating cancer is that the immune system does not recognize the cancerous cells as the enemy. Instead of attacking tumor cells, the immune system's defenses treat them as a natural part of the body. With the prostate cancer vaccine, specialized white blood cells called dendritic cells are drawn from the body and treated in the laboratory so that they become sensitive to malignant cells. Then the dendritic cells are injected back into the body, where they launch an attack on the cancer.

Clinical trials of the therapy are going on across the country with some success. A 1998 study from researchers at Northwest Hospital's Pacific Northwest Cancer Foundation looked at 33 patients with advanced prostate cancer that was unresponsive to other therapies. Nine of the men in the study (27 percent) had

continues

> either a 50 percent reduction in PSA levels or a decrease of 50 percent or more in tumor size with no progression elsewhere. Another 11 men (33 percent) showed stable disease.
>
> The vaccine is currently being designed for use by men with advanced prostate cancer that hasn't responded to other forms of treatment and by those whose prostate cancer has returned after being treated. Eventually, however, researchers hope the vaccine will become a primary form of treatment for the disease.

As with any cancer, men with prostate cancer have sought and tried miracle "cures," including vitamins and fad foods; one urged on Cornelius Ryan, as he recounted in *A Private Battle,* was Eskimo soup made from the blood and guts of various animals.

A macrobiotic diet is also sometimes used to help fight prostate cancer or cancer in general. One case you may have heard of involved Anthony J. Sattilaro, the Philadelphia physician and president of Methodist Hospital, who was diagnosed with metastatic prostate cancer in 1978, at the age of 47. Sattilaro, who received a bilateral orchiectomy and hormonal treatment, tried a macrobiotic diet and felt it helped him so much that he promoted it widely.

A macrobiotic diet consists primarily of whole grains like brown rice, along with some vegetables, beans, and seaweed. It excludes all meat, dairy products, sugar, oils, and synthetic chemicals and preservatives. It's designed for an individual and adjusted on a seasonal basis.

By 1982, when Sattilaro completed his book, *Recalled by Life,* and gave the diet wide publicity, his cancer was in total remission. Ultimately, he died of prostate cancer, but not until 1989, 11 years after his initial diagnosis.

This doesn't prove that a macrobiotic diet helped Sattilaro. Cancer specialists believe that his improvement was due to the surgery and additional hormone treatment. In fact, some doctors say a macrobiotic diet can actually be harmful because it's low in vitamins and minerals that people need and doesn't allow vitamin and mineral supplements.

Watchful Waiting

The term *nontreatment* is something of a misnomer. Patients who choose not to be treated may still receive hormonal therapy if their tumors progress and they develop symptoms. That's why "watchful waiting" may be a more precise description of what actually takes place.

A number of studies support the concept of watchful waiting. In 1992, researchers in Sweden published a landmark study of 642 men with untreated early prostate cancer. The average age at diagnosis was 72. Of the men, 223 were assigned to a deferred treatment group (meaning they were not treated until symptoms appeared), while 77 were treated aggressively from the start. A 10-year follow-up showed the deferred group had survival rates similar to those who received standard intervention—either radical prostatectomy or radiation. The survival rates were still the same in both groups at the time of a 15-year follow-up, published by the same researchers in 1997.

This study showed that a man can choose nontreatment and have the same survival rate as a man treated aggressively (who must also deal with potential side effects). That's certainly one conclusion, although the results should be viewed as cautiously as any other research findings. For example, Joseph Oesterling, M.D., of the Mayo Clinic, has remarked that most of the men in the Swedish study were older and had a shorter life expectancy than would be the case for men with diagnosed cancer as part of a large-scale screening program in the United States.

Unfortunately, there aren't any comparable studies on men under the age of 60. But one study that otherwise gave strong support for a "wait-and-see" approach did offer some support for intervention in certain cases. Published in the *Journal of the American Medical Association* in 1993, the research looked at men ages 60 to 75 years with stages T1 and T2 prostate cancer. The researchers reported that those who were 60 to 65 years old did benefit from treatment such as prostatectomy or radiation if their tumors were relatively aggressive.

For this study, the Prostate Patient Outcomes Research Team, which includes researchers from a number of medical establishments, measured the benefit of treatment in terms of "quality-adjusted life expectancy"—"quality" being an aggregate measure of impotence, incontinence, and other complications of both cancer and its treatment. The study found that relatively younger men with faster-growing localized tumors could gain up to 3.5 years in quality-adjusted life expectancy if they chose a radical prostatectomy or radiation therapy over watchful waiting.

The marginal benefit of treatment, however, dipped sharply—to less than a year—when the tumor was slow growing. For older men, the gain in quality-adjusted life expectancy was less than six months. And for some patients, nontreatment was clearly preferable to treatment.

For T3 stage tumors, there is little information on the impact that watchful waiting or treatment may have. But a study by researchers at the Memorial Sloan-Kettering Cancer Center did look into nontreatment in the case of 35 men with newly diagnosed metastasized prostate cancer but with minimal symptoms of disease. It compared the quality of life of patients who received hormonal therapy when they were diagnosed, with that of men who decided to defer treatment until their PSA levels or symptoms worsened. (In this case, "quality of life" included such elements as the patients' social life, feelings of well-being and anxiety, and independence.)

Researchers found that the group that opted for deferred treatment had fewer sexual problems and more physical energy than the group that had hormonal therapy. After six months, the group being treated was suffering more psychological distress. Concerning the group that chose not to be treated, the researchers wrote, "Quality of survival was equally important to overall survival time."

Survival itself wasn't an issue in the study. The data were drawn from questionnaires completed by the patients themselves over a period of six months after they made their initial decision about treatment.

You would think nontreatment to be without complications, but they do occur. Urinary obstruction can be said to be a side effect of nontreatment if the tumor remains localized. In one study, approximately one-third of patients required at least one transurethral prostatectomy, or TURP, the procedure we describe in Chapter 4, for the relief of bladder outlet obstructions. However, it's not entirely certain that cancer growth was responsible for the obstructions.

Although TURP is an option for cancer patients, studies have connected it to an increase in metastasis and a decrease in survival for patients whose cancer hasn't yet metastasized at the time they have the procedure. Researchers have found they can reduce the risk somewhat by lowering the pressure they use in irrigating. (During a TURP, the surgical area is regularly flushed with fluid to keep it clear of blood.)

In a recent article in *Ca,* the American Cancer Society's publication for clinicians, two physicians who looked at this problem conclude that, if TURP is absolutely necessary to relieve a patient's obstruction, his doctor should consider radiating the tumor once to reduce both its size and the likelihood that it would spread during the procedure.

In addition to the various side effects we describe in Chapter 4, TURP may have potentially more severe complications when prostate cancer is involved. As the prostate becomes filled with tumor, the prostatic urethra turns into a rigid tube. As a result, about 5 percent of patients who have TURP to relieve obstructions from advanced prostatic cancer develop incontinence problems.

Severe bleeding during a TURP can also be a greater problem than with BPH patients, because certain substances in the cancerous tissue promote bleeding and prevent blood clotting.

For someone with prostate cancer, alternatives to TURP include transrectal microwave hyperthermia, the heat therapy we describe in Chapter 4. One recent study found that transrectal microwave hyperthermia is actually more effective in relieving bladder obstruction in men with prostate cancer than in men who have only BPH. The researchers report that five weeks of heat therapy led to relief over the following two years, and 80 percent of the subjects reported an improvement in quality of life.

Choosing Your Treatment According to Stage

You must make your decision regarding which form of treatment that is best for you in consultation with your doctor and family. If you consult with more than one doctor, you may hear more than one opinion. As we said earlier, there's considerable disagreement within medical circles about which treatments are most effective.

But what we can tell you in this section are the most common treatments for each stage, as indicated by the National Cancer Institute. Note the wide range of options. In each case, however, you should keep in mind that nontreatment, or watchful waiting, is always an option, regardless of your age or health.

The treatment of stage T1 cancer depends on how much of the prostate is affected. If only a small number of cancer cells are found and if you're older, your doctor may follow you closely without any treatment. She may choose this option for you because your cancer is not causing any symptoms or other problems and may be growing slowly.

If cancer cells can be detected microscopically in many areas of the prostate, your treatment may be one of the following:

1. External radiation therapy

2. Radical prostatectomy, usually with pelvic lymph node dissection. Radiation therapy may be given after surgery in some cases.

In the Lab: Getting Involved in Clinical Trials

Clinical trials for new treatments, as well as for different combinations of established therapies, are going on in most parts of the country, for most stages of prostate cancer. As this section reveals, clinical trials are among the treatment options for men with prostate cancer.

A clinical trial is an organized study that aims to answer specific questions about a new treatment or a new approach to a known treatment. For example, a trial might look at the effectiveness of an anticancer drug, the benefits and risks of a surgical procedure, or how a change in diet or lifestyle affects a person's condition.

Clinical trials—which are performed with people only after the treatment in question is studied in a laboratory and in animals—help researchers develop new treatments that are safe and effective—treatments that could save lives. People with cancer often get involved with trials both to have the opportunity to try a new form of treatment and to help others with cancer by contributing to research.

If you are thinking of joining a trial, the National Cancer Institute recommends asking the following questions:

- What is the purpose of the study?
- What does the study involve? What sort of tests and treatments are offered? How are they performed?

continues

- What will happen to my condition with or without the experimental treatment? What is it expected to do?
- What are the advantages and disadvantages of the study? (While you may receive an experimental treatment, for example, you may be required to follow a strict diet or forgo another form of treatment.)
- How will the study affect my daily life?
- What side effects can I expect from the study?
- How long will the study last?
- Will I need to go to the hospital? If so, for how long?
- What costs are involved in the study? What will I pay, and what will the study pay?
- Will I be entitled to any treatment if I'm harmed as a result of the study?
- Will any long-term follow-up care be involved in the study?

If you're interested in participating in such research, talk to your doctor or contact the National Cancer Institute (NCI) at the listing shown at the end of this book to determine if you are eligible. NCI's computerized resource of cancer treatment information, PDQ, has an up-to-date list of clinical trials in progress all over the country.

Treatment of Prostate Cancer

3. Interstitial radiation therapy, often using ultrasound or CT guidance to place the implants
4. Nontreatment, if you are older or have another, more serious illness. In this case, your doctor may follow you closely without treatment.
5. A clinical trial of external radiation therapy using new techniques to protect your normal tissues from radiation

If you have stage T2 cancer, which is still contained within the prostate and is typically detected during a routine rectal exam, your treatment may be one of the following:

1. Radical prostatectomy, usually with pelvic lymph node dissection. Radiation therapy may be given following surgery.
2. External radiation therapy
3. Interstitial radiation therapy, often using ultrasound or CT guidance to place the implants
4. Nontreatment, if you are older or have another more serious illness. Your doctor may choose this option for you because your cancer is not causing any symptoms or other problems and may be growing slowly.
5. A clinical trial of external radiation therapy using new techniques to protect your normal tissues from radiation. Other clinical trials are testing new types of radiation.

6. A clinical trial of ultrasound-guided cryosurgery

In the case of stage T3 cancer, which is still localized but may extend beyond the prostatic capsule to involve the seminal vesicles as well, your treatment may be one of the following:

1. Hormonal manipulations (removal of the testicles or use of LHRH analogs or estrogen)

2. External radiation therapy

3. Radical prostatectomy and usually pelvic lymph node dissection. Radiation therapy may be given following surgery.

4. Nontreatment, if you are older or have another more serious illness. Your doctor may choose this option for you because your cancer is not causing any symptoms or other problems and may be growing slowly.

If you're unable to undergo surgery or radiation therapy, your doctor may give you treatments to relieve symptoms, such as problems urinating. In this case, your treatment may be one of the following:

1. Radiation therapy to relieve symptoms

2. Hormone manipulations (removal of the testicles or use of LHRH analogs or estrogen)

3. TURP

4. Interstitial radiation therapy combined with external mean radiation therapy

5. Clinical trials using alternative forms of radiotherapy, such as proton therapy

6. Clinical trials of ultrasound-guided cryosurgery

With stage T4, your treatment depends on how far the cancer has spread from the prostate. Your treatment may be one of the following:

1. Hormone manipulations (removal of the testicles or use of LHRH analogs or estrogen)

2. External radiation therapy, including clinical trials for new forms of radiation. Hormone therapy may be given in addition to radiation. Radiation may also be done simply to relieve symptoms.

3. Radical prostatectomy and orchiectomy

4. Nontreatment, if you are older or have another more serious illness. Your doctor may choose this option for you because your cancer is not causing any symptoms or other problems and may be growing slowly.

5. TURP (to help relieve symptoms only)

6. Clinical trials of system chemotherapy

If the tumor recurs, your treatment depends on many things, including what treatment you had before. If you had a radical prostatectomy and the cancer comes back in only a small area, you may receive radiation therapy. If the disease has spread to other parts of your body, you will probably undergo hormone therapy. Radiation therapy may be given as well, to relieve symptoms such as bone pain. You may also choose to take part in a clinical trial of chemotherapy or biological therapy.

Follow-Up

Whatever treatment—or nontreatment—you choose, you'll have regular follow-up exams to monitor your condition. If the cancer was confined to the prostate, your doctor will want to make sure that it hasn't returned. If it has spread beyond the prostate, you should be examined to see what other medical care is necessary. Your doctor will determine how often to schedule these exams.

The doctor will want to know whether you've had any changes in appetite, any urinary problems, dramatic weight fluctuations, or bone pain, all of which could indicate metastasis. We discuss many of the tests and procedures elsewhere in this book because they're also diagnostic tools.

To keep tabs on your condition, the doctor should perform a rectal exam to check for new nodules. He'll run a PSA test. PSA levels should be undetectable unless disease remains. In fact, the PSA test was first used to confirm the success of a radical prostatectomy, and it is currently felt to be very helpful in determining the risk for cancer recurrence. There'll be a urinalysis and possibly other blood tests to determine if your liver and kidneys are functioning properly.

You may have an annual bone scan and bone x-ray to see whether the cancer has spread. If you have prostatic bleeding, which shows up in your urine, your doctor might use a cystoscope to locate its source and also to assess the degree of obstruction to urine flow caused by the tumor.

Recurrence

If your practitioner finds that the cancer has spread, you'll be treated for any symptoms and side effects caused by the metastatic tumor itself. These symptoms will be different for each patient, depending on the location of the metastasis. Some of the more common problems are due to metastasis to bones, especially the spine or skull, or to the brain.

If the growing tumor presses on the spinal cord, it can cause a condition called spinal cord compression; symptoms include back pain, muscle weakness, decreased sensation, and loss of bowel or bladder function. This is a medical emergency that must be treated immediately to reduce the risk of permanent neurological injury. Usually, the patient receives medication, followed by either radiation or surgery.

If the tumor metastasizes to the skull or brain, headache, seizures, or other neurological problems may develop. Like the problems caused by spinal cord compression, these are also emergency conditions that require immediate medical attention.

Pain management can be an important part of care for men with prostate cancer. Depending on the metastasis, your doctor may use radiation, hormonal therapy, or other approaches to shrink the tumor.

The trouble is that the treatments themselves can produce other problems. Radiation therapy directed to the base of the skull, for example, can produce irreversible neurologic injury, and the pain relief is temporary.

Recently, there has been some interest in **radiopharmaceuticals** such as strontium-89, a radioactive element that is given by vein and builds up in high concentrations in metastases within bone. These drugs may be less toxic than external radiation and relieve pain significantly. However, they're no substitute for conventional radiation therapy in preventing spinal cord compression.

Doctors also use anti-inflammatory drugs in combination with morphine to treat pain. Keep in mind that not all drugs are equally effective against all cancers; what works for metastatic bone pain from breast cancer, for example, may not be effective against metastatic bone pain from prostate cancer.

Metastases to the hip and pelvis often produce local pain that's exacerbated by movement, especially during weight-bearing movement. In addition to radiation therapy, your doctor may try to control the pain through orthopedic measures, such as pinning and otherwise stabilizing the bone.

If your cancer resists therapy, you may want to consider, and discuss with your family and physician, issues regarding quality of life versus measures to prolong life.

If you decide you don't want to treat the tumor further, your doctor can suggest ways that you can receive symptomatic relief and support outside the hospital. In the past decade, there's been a tremendous development of facilities and techniques that allow you to remain in your home. A vast home-health infrastructure can provide comprehensive nursing care and supervision, as well as psychological support.

Alternatively, you may wish to participate in cancer treatment trials of drugs or other approaches that are highly experimental and of unknown benefit. You can ask NCI or your doctor to put you in touch with large cancer centers that are running such trials.

The Emotional Effects of Cancer Treatment

It's easy to get caught up in the statistics and studies surrounding prostate cancer and forget about the immense emotional impact the condition can have on a man. Being diagnosed with any form of cancer is difficult—you might have concerns not only about death, but also about issues such as scarring, pain, and changes in employment and lifestyle. In addition, prostate cancer carries with it the specter of impotence and incontinence—complications that may be difficult to cope with in and of themselves.

DIGESTING THE DIAGNOSIS

There's plenty of information out there, and in this book, about prostate cancer. You'll find mortality rates and survival rates, as well as details about specific treatments and their side effects. But information on coping with cancer is more difficult to find. After all, emotions aren't often the subject of studies on prostate cancer.

One thing is for sure: There's no such thing as a wrong reaction to being told you have cancer. Anger, sadness, frustration, fear, and courage are just a few of the emotions a man may experience when he is first told he has cancer. These emotions can be complicated by the fact that the announcement might come after days of anxiety and worry over pending test results.

Even when the initial shock has passed, adjusting to the idea of having cancer is difficult—and different people handle the news in different ways. Some wish to remain close-mouthed about it and resist sharing their feelings with family and friends.

Others may share their feelings openly. All reactions are normal. But it's important to remember that, for most people, the outlook for prostate cancer is a positive one. Although every case is different and there are no guarantees, there are good possibilities for the future.

One caveat: The first days after receiving a diagnosis can be the most trying. Not only are you trying to cope with bad news, but you're also faced with a landslide of information and a host of treatment options. To make sure you get all the facts, take a trusted friend or family member—or a tape recorder, for that matter—with you to your doctor's appointment. That way, if you miss a crucial piece of information or can't quite remember what was said, you'll be able to double-check the facts with the person who was with you. Another person can also help by asking questions or requesting clarification if you're unable to do so yourself.

COPING WITH CANCER

To help you come to terms with cancer, experts offer the following advice:

- Become well-informed about your condition and its effects. The information will help put you at ease—after all, the unknown is much more frightening than the known—and will also help you become an active partner in your own health care.

- Talk frankly with your doctor. Find out what you can expect both from the cancer and from the treatment. The more information you have, the easier it is to make the choices that are right for you.

- Speak up. As you become more familiar with your treatment, you may be able to work with your doctor in planning your treatment regimen. If you feel that a different diet or dosage of medication will work better for you—perhaps help you avoid some side effects—let your physician know.

- Keep lines of communication open. It may be difficult for you to talk about your prostate cancer to others, and others may feel uncomfortable talking about it with you. However, sharing your anxieties and feelings can help make coping with cancer easier. Meeting with a member of the clergy, a counselor, or another outside party may help.

- Take it easy. It may be difficult to keep up with an already busy schedule once you learn you have cancer. What's more, trying to do too much can make healing more difficult. Give yourself permission to cut back on activities and social events. You may also want to consider hiring a housekeeper or maintenance service to keep up your house or yard.

- Change doctors if you're not getting the information and support you need. If your doctor doesn't provide you with all of the facts or is too busy or inattentive to address your concerns, think about finding a new practitioner. In order to receive the best treatment possible, you need to find a doctor who will be a partner in your care.

- Practice a relaxation technique. Stress is a natural accompaniment to any serious health condition, and—if it gets out of hand—it can take its own toll on the body by raising heart and blood pressure rates, among other things. To help fight stress, practice breathing deeply, visualize a peaceful scene, or perform a yoga routine.

THE VALUE OF SUPPORT GROUPS

Talking about prostate cancer can be a difficult proposition because the condition affects the reproductive system—a sensitive subject—and because it may lead to what many feel are embarrassing side effects: impotence and incontinence.

Support groups overcome these obstacles to communication by providing a forum in which people with cancer can share information, emotions, and experiences. While at one time such groups were dismissed as "pity-parties," they are now considered to be an important part of the cancer treatment program. In fact, researchers believe emotional support can even strengthen the body's defenses against cancer.

In 1989, for example, a Stanford study of women with metastatic breast cancer found that those who participated in support groups were less anxious, less depressed, and had less pain than those who did not participate. What's even more impressive, however, is that a four-year follow-up found that the women in the support group lived an average of 18 months longer than the others.

A 1990 study from the University of California had similar results. People with malignant melanoma who participated in group counseling reported less stress and an easier time coping than those who didn't participate. Participants also had an increase in the number of natural killer cells—immune system cells that are capable of destroying cancerous tumor cells. Five years later, those in the support group had significantly better survival rates than those who didn't attend.

Support groups give people with cancer an opportunity to share practical information, such as knowledge of new treatments or opinions on doctors in the area. But they also allow for a release of damaging stress by giving people a chance to talk about their fears and worries—problems that well-meaning friends and family members without cancer might not understand. Support groups can also provide self-confidence and feelings of hope for the future.

A number of support groups are available for men with prostate cancer. Ask your practitioner about groups in your local area.

The one national group, Man to Man, is organized by the American Cancer Society. It offers group education and support, personal visitation and telephone support, quarterly newsletters, awareness activities, educational materials, and an Internet Web site. Another group, US TOO, provides those with prostate cancer with emotional and educational support through a network of support groups. They also offer a quarterly newsletter. An on-line search or a trip to the library may also turn up groups in your area.

CANCER AND DEPRESSION

Naturally, a diagnosis of cancer leads to feelings of sadness and loss. But clinical depression is more than just a passing blue mood. Depression consists of sadness, hopelessness, a general disinterest in life, and a sense of reduced emotional well-being. Unlike the occasional sadness that most people experience, depression deepens and is persistent. It becomes a true depressive illness when it affects a person's behavior and physical state, often leading to insomnia, digestive problems, sore muscles, headaches, and backaches.

For those with cancer, depression may be brought on by a change or loss in life, hormonal changes, the cancer itself, and even some cancer drugs. Signs of depression include changing your eating habits, sleeping too much or too little, gaining or losing large amounts of weight, and experiencing long-lasting feelings of sadness.

If you're suffering from depression, don't expect to "snap out of it" on your own. Depression is a serious condition and may require counseling or other mental health services. Through such services, people can help get over feelings of anxiety, sadness, and hopelessness and learn how to cope with their conditions. Your primary care practitioner can refer you to a specialist in mental health if necessary.

Having a prostate problem isn't easy—whether it's cancer, benign prostatic hyperplasia, or a case of prostatitis. It is hoped that this book has made it easier by giving you the information you need to make informed decisions about your health care. By knowing about prostate disease and its symptoms, diagnosis, and treatment, you're in a better position to make the right choices for yourself.

Informational and Mutual-Aid Groups

Agency for Health Care Policy and Research Publications Clearinghouse
P.O. Box 8547
Silver Spring, MD 20907-8547
800-358-9295
www.ahcpr.gov

American Cancer Society
1599 Clifton Rd., N.E.
Atlanta, GA 30329-4251
800-ACS-2345
(check your phone book for a local ACS office)
www.cancer.org

American Foundation for Urologic Disease Bladder Health Council
300 W. Pratt St., Suite 401
Baltimore, MD 21201
800-242-2383

American Urological Association
1120 N. Charles St.
Baltimore, MD 21201
410-727-1100

ChemoCare
231 North Ave., W.
Westfield, NJ 07090-1428
800-55-CHEMO
908-233-1103 (in New Jersey)

Chemotherapy Foundation
183 Madison Ave., Suite 403
New York, NY 10016
212-213-9292

Impotence World Institute
P.O. Box 410
Bowie, MD 20718-0410
800-669-1603

Man to Man
800-ACS-2345
www.cancer.org

Mathews Foundation for Prostate Cancer Research
817 Commons Dr.
Sacramento, CA 95825
800-234-6284
916-567-1400

National Association for Continence
P.O. Box 8310
Spartenburg, SC 29305
800-BLADDER
www.nafc.org

National Cancer Institute
National Institutes of Health
9000 Rockville Pike
Bethesda, MD 20892
800-4-CANCER
www.cancernet.nci.nih.gov

National Institute on Aging Information Center
P.O. Box 8057
Gaithersburg, MD 20898-8057
800-222-2225
www.nih.gov/nia

National Kidney and Urologic Diseases Information Clearinghouse
3 Information Way
Bethesda, MD 20892-3580
www.aerie.com/nihdb/nkudic/kudbase.html

Patient Advocates for Advanced Cancer Treatments (PAACT)
P.O. Box 141695
Grand Rapids, MI 49514
616-453-1477
www.osz.com/paact

Prostate Health Council
c/o American Foundation for Urologic Disease, Inc.
1128 N. Charles St.
Baltimore, MD 21201-5559
800-242-2383
www.afud.org

The Simon Foundation
P.O. Box 815
Wilmette, IL 60091
800-23-SIMON
www.incontinet.com
(for incontinence)

US TOO International
930 N. York Rd., St. 50
Hinsdale, IL 60521-2993
800-80-US-TOO
www.ustoo.com

Glossary

Acute bacterial prostatitis   A rare and serious prostatic disease that results from a sudden infusion of bacteria into the prostate.

Acute urinary retention   A condition, sometimes triggered by alcohol, cold, immobility, or certain medications, in which a man suddenly finds himself completely unable to urinate.

Adjuvant   Treatment that is offered after the most effective form of therapy has been tried.

Alpha-adrenergic blockers   A group of drugs that relax the smooth muscle tissue in both the prostate and the bladder neck, thus easing constriction of the urethra.

Analgesics   Pain-relief medications.

Androgens   A class of male hormones.

Antiandrogen   A drug that, as part of hormonal therapy, blocks the effect of any remaining androgens.

Antihypertensive   Blood-pressure-lowering medication that, because it also relaxes muscles, is sometimes prescribed for benign prostatic hyperplasia.

Glossary

Anus The opening of the rectum where solid waste leaves the body.

Aromatase An enzyme that converts testosterone into the form of estrogen that is found in men and is thought to contribute to BPH.

Artificial insemination A reproductive technique in which sperm is extracted from a man after ejaculation and then deposited in a woman's vagina.

Artificial urinary sphincter A device designed to restore control to an incontinent person by giving him the mechanical means of opening and closing his urethra.

Aspiration The removal of fluids by suction, often through a needle that is attached to a syringe.

Bacterial prostatitis Prostatitis, or inflammation of the prostate, caused by bacteria.

Balloon dilatation *See* **Balloon urethroplasty.**

Balloon urethroplasty (or Balloon dilatation) A balloon treatment of the urethra to compress the prostate and widen the urethra, easing the flow of urine.

Benign Noncancerous.

Benign prostatic hyperplasia (BPH) A noncancerous enlargement of the prostate through the multiplication of the number of cells. Occurring mainly in elderly men, the overgrowth of prostate tissue may push against the urethra and the bladder, blocking the flow of urine and causing acute discomfort.

Beta carotene A compound, found in foods, that can be converted in the body to an active form of vitamin A.

Bilateral orchiectomy　A procedure in which both testes are removed, generally through an incision in the scrotal bag, to eliminate the main source of male hormones and slow the spread of prostate cancer.

Biofeedback　A technique in which a person learns to consciously control involuntary responses, such as muscle contractions, by having these responses initially monitored electronically.

Biopsy　Removal of a small tissue sample for microscopic examination.

Bladder　The hollow organ in the lower abdomen where urine is stored.

Bladder catheterization　A diagnostic or therapeutic procedure in which a thin rubber tube is inserted up the urethra into the bladder.

Blood-prostate barrier　The portion of the prostate that prevents certain substances from entering and effectively keeps out most antibiotics, making it difficult to treat infections.

Bone scan　A highly sensitive process that uses a radioactive substance to image the bone structure.

Brachytherapy (or Interstitial radiation therapy)　Internal radiation therapy, generated by radioactive material implanted as "seeds" or "pellets" in and around the cancerous area, such as in the prostate.

Carotenoid　Any of a group of red, yellow, or orange pigments found in foods such as carrots, sweet potatoes, and leafy green vegetables. The body converts this substance to vitamin A.

Catheter　A tubular medical device inserted into a canal, vessel, passageway, or body cavity, usually used to inject or withdraw fluids or to keep a passage open.

Glossary

Cellule A small pouch that develops between trabeculations.

Chlamydia The most common sexually transmitted disease, a bacterial infection acquired chiefly through vaginal or anal intercourse.

Chronic bacterial prostatitis A recurring bacterial infection in the prostate.

Coitus interruptus The interruption of sexual intercourse, generally for contraceptive purposes, to enable the man to ejaculate outside the vagina.

Colon bacilli Bacteria that are in the colon.

Compensated bladder A bladder that empties completely on voiding.

Computerized tomography (CT or CAT) scan A series of detailed pictures of areas inside the body, created by a computer linked to an x-ray machine.

Congestive prostatitis *See* **Prostatostasis**.

Creatinine A metabolic waste product, the blood level of which is an important measure of kidney function.

Cryosurgery A surgical procedure employing liquid nitrogen at exceptionally low temperatures to freeze and destroy tissue.

Curative Potentially capable of completely destroying a cancer.

Cystoscopy A procedure in which a cystoscope—a slender, hollow tube with a lens at each end—is passed into the penile urethra and bladder, allowing visual examination of the urinary tract.

Decompensated bladder A bladder that does not empty completely on voiding, so that residual urine remains.

Digital (manual) rectal exam A procedure in which a doctor inserts a gloved, lubricated finger into the rectum and, through the wall of the rectum, checks the prostate for hard or lumpy areas.

Dihydrotestosterone (DHT) A more active form of testosterone that tends to be highly concentrated in the prostate and has been implicated in the benign enlargement of the prostate.

Diverticula Pouches or sacs that branch out from the bladder when the bladder muscle is overworked.

Dry orgasm *See* **Retrograde ejaculation**.

Epididymis An elongated, cordlike structure in the testes that stores and transmits sperm.

Epididymitis Inflammation of the epididymis.

Estrogen A female hormone.

Excretory urogram (or Intravenous pyelogram [IVP] or Intravenous urogram [IVUI]) A test performed by the injection of a dye that concentrates in the kidneys. A series of x-rays are then taken at timed intervals to provide information about the entire urinary tract, including size of the prostate, size of the bladder, and kidney functioning.

External-beam radiotherapy Radiation therapy delivered from a machine, either a lower-voltage cobalt unit or a higher-voltage linear accelerator.

Fistula An abnormal connection between two hollow spaces or organs.

5-alpha-reductase An enzyme that converts testosterone into a more active androgen called dihydrotestosterone.

Glossary

Foley catheter A catheter that is placed into the bladder for continuous drainage and left in place by means of a liquid-filled balloon within the bladder.

Gland An aggregation of cells, specialized to secrete or excrete materials.

Gonorrhea A sexually transmitted bacterial infection that may involve the urethra.

Growth factors Proteins that may act on tissue to cause enlargements, such as benign prostatic hyperplasia.

Hematuria Blood or red blood cells in the urine.

Hesitancy The condition when a man has to wait for several seconds to a couple of minutes for his urine flow to start while the bladder muscle strains against the resistance of the prostate.

Hormonal therapy The use of medications or the surgical removal of the testicles to prevent male hormones from stimulating further growth of prostate cancer.

Hyperthermia *See* **Thermotherapy.**

Impotence The inability of a male to develop or maintain an erection sufficient to copulate.

Incontinence A person's inability to control urination.

Intermittency An involuntary stopping and starting of the urinary stream.

Interstitial radiation therapy *See* **Brachytherapy.**

Intravenous pyelogram (IVP) *See* **Excretory urogram.**

Intravenous urogram (IVU) *See* **Excretory urogram.**

Laparoscopy   The use of small tubes to gain access to the interior of the abdomen. In a laparoscopic pelvic lymph node dissection, a doctor can remove and examine lymph nodes.

Luteinizing hormone-releasing hormone (LHRH) analog   A laboratory-made substance that works against LHRH, which is a hormone that normally controls the production of sex hormones, to eliminate or slow the spread of cancer.

Lymphadenectomy   A biopsy of the lymph nodes.

Lymphangiogram   An imaging procedure in which dye is injected into the lymph system and travels to the pelvic area, concentrating in such a way that an x-ray can reveal cancer in the nodes.

Lymph nodes   Small glands located in many areas of the body that help defend the body against harmful foreign particles. Prostate cancer often spreads first to the pelvic lymph nodes.

Magnetic resonance imaging (MRI)   An imaging technique that produces detailed pictures of areas inside the body by linking a computer with a powerful magnet.

Metastasize   Spread, as in the case of cancer, to distant organs or tissues.

Nafarelin acetate   A hormone blocker that inhibits the testes' production of testosterone by acting on the pituitary gland.

Necrosis   The death of living tissue.

Nocturia   The urge or need to urinate at night.

Nonbacterial prostatitis   *See* **Prostatodynia** and **Prostatostasis**.

Nonspecific urethritis (NSU)   An infection of the prostatic urethra.

Glossary

Palliative Capable of reducing the symptoms of a disease and slowing its growth, but unable to wipe it out.

Perineum In a man, the area between the scrotum and the anus.

Prostate A walnut-size gland in the male reproductive system that surrounds part of the urethra and secretes most of the fluid that is ejaculated with sperm during orgasm.

Prostate cancer A malignant and hence potentially serious disease of the prostate that accounts for more deaths in men than any other cancer except skin cancer.

Prostatectomy *See* **Transurethral resection of the prostate (TURP)** and **Radical prostatectomy**.

Prostate-specific antigen (PSA) A substance, produced exclusively by prostate cells, whose level increases in the presence of prostatic cancer and rises significantly with metastasis, or spread, of the cancer.

Prostatic acid phosphatase (PAP) Another substance produced by prostate cells. An increase in PAP indicates the spread of prostate cancer.

Prostatic urethra The portion of the urethra that is within the prostate.

Prostatitis An inflammation of the prostate, which may or may not be caused by the presence of bacteria.

Prostatodynia A form of nonbacterial prostatitis, in which pain seems to be coming from the prostate but is much more likely to be coming from the muscles of the floor of the pelvis, from an inflammation in one or more of the pelvic bones, or from a disease in the rectum.

Prostatostasis (or Congestive prostatitis) The most common form of nonbacterial prostatitis, generally attributed to the accumulation of excess fluid within the prostate.

Prosthesis A device that, surgically implanted within the body, replicates natural body functions or parts. A penile prosthesis allows an impotent man to have erections for intercourse.

Radiation therapy The use of high-energy rays to shrink tumors and stop cancer cells from growing. Like surgery, it is local therapy, affecting only the cells in the treated area.

Radical prostatectomy The complete surgical removal of the prostate, usually for prostatic cancer.

Radiopharmaceuticals Radioactive drugs used for diagnostic or therapeutic purposes.

Rectum The portion of the large intestine between the colon and the anus.

Reflux A potentially dangerous condition in which, because of prostatic growth, urine is unable to leave the bladder through the urethra and eventually backs up into the kidneys.

Renal scan An image of the kidneys produced by injecting radioactive material.

Resectoscope The instrument, used in a TURP, that allows the surgeon to resect, or cut, and remove the obstructing prostatic tissue.

Retrograde ejaculation Male orgasm without the release of seminal fluid through the penis.

Retropubic The area behind and below the pubic bone.

Scrotum The sac of skin that contains the testicles.

Segmented urine culture A series of tests, typically to check for prostatitis, in which the person urinates at intervals into three separate cups.

Seminal vesicles The two saclike structures directly behind the base of the bladder that contribute to the production of semen.

Silent prostatism An infrequent condition in which a man may be unaware he has a urinary obstruction until he suddenly becomes completely unable to urinate. Untreated, the condition leads to kidney failure, coma, and death.

Sonogram An image obtained by ultrasonic scanning.

Spermatozoa The male reproductive cells.

Staging The effort to determine whether a cancer has spread and what parts of the body are involved.

Stent A stainless-steel device that can be inserted semipermanently into the prostatic urethra to stretch it and let urine flow more easily.

Stress incontinence Involuntary release of urine when there is an increase in pressure within the bladder, usually from coughing, laughing, or straining.

Stricture Abnormal narrowing of a bodily passage, often by scarring.

Stroma The tissue framework, as distinguished from the specific substance, of an organ or gland.

Suprapubic Above the pubic bone.

Sympathomimetic A decongestant drug that may, as a side effect, tighten the bladder neck and make it difficult to urinate.

Systemic Pervading the entire body rather than being limited to an area or organ. Systemic therapy reaches cancer cells throughout the body.

Testicles The male glands that produce sperm and male hormones.

Testosterone A male hormone produced mainly by the testicles.

Thermotherapy The application of microwave heat to the enlarged prostate with the object of shrinking or destroying the BPH tissue.

Trabeculation Irregular bands of thickened muscle tissue that develop in the bladder wall as the prostate enlarges and the bladder muscle has to work harder to force out urine.

Transrectal microwave hyperthermia A procedure in which heat is applied to the prostate by means of a microwave probe inserted through the rectum, to relieve the condition known as BPH.

Transrectal ultrasonography An examination that produces an image of the prostate by inserting a probe into the rectum to direct sound waves to the prostate.

Transurethral hyperthermia Same as transrectal microwave hyperthermia, but with the probe inserted through the urethra.

Transurethral incision of the prostate (TUIP) A more limited version of TURP, in which a surgeon makes two incisions from the bladder neck through the prostate to widen the urinary passage but does not resect the enlarged prostate.

Transurethral microwave thermotherapy (TUMT) A procedure to relieve the condition known as BPH, in which a modified Foley catheter containing a microwave antenna is inserted through the urethra and heats the tissues deep within the prostate.

Transurethral resection of the prostate (TURP) The most common procedure for BPH, in which a surgeon tunnels through the urethra with a resectoscope to cut away the enlarged tissue.

Transurethral ultrasound-guided laser-induced prostatectomy (TULIP) A highly experimental procedure to destroy BPH tissue by inserting a laser probe into the urethra and an ultrasound probe in the rectum to direct the laser energy, which superheats and destroys the tissue.

Ultrasonic aspiration A highly experimental procedure to improve urine flow in men with BPH by directing ultrasound vibrations against the enlarged portion of the prostate and "disrupting" the tissue. The tissue is then aspirated through the device.

Ultrasound A procedure that bounces high-frequency sound waves off tissues and converts the echoes into images.

Urea nitrogen A waste product whose presence in the blood is used to measure kidney function.

Uremic poisoning (or Uremia) A condition arising from kidney failure, which can lead to unconsciousness and death.

Ureters The two very thin, muscular tubes that transport urine from the kidneys to the bladder.

Urethra The canal inside the penis through which urine and semen pass as they leave the body.

Urethral sphincter The muscle located just beyond the prostate, enclosing part of the urethra, that a man voluntarily contracts to shut off his urinary flow.

Urinalysis The physical, chemical, and microscopic analysis of urine for abnormalities.

Urinary retention   A condition in which some urine remains in the bladder, because of a constricted urethra, even after a man has voided.

Urine culture   The incubation of urine at a specific temperature so as to permit the growth and identification of microorganisms.

Urodynamic studies   Quantitative analysis of the two principal functions of the bladder, urine storage and voiding.

Uroflometer   A machine used to conduct a urodynamic evaluation by measuring the rate of urine flow.

Urologist   A physician specializing in diseases of the urinary tract and the male reproductive system.

Vas deferens   The two tubes that carry the sperm from the testes to the urethra.

Vasectomy   An operation, generally for contraceptive purposes, in which the vas deferens are sealed off.

Suggested Reading

Baggish, Jeff. *Making the Prostate Therapy Decision.* Los Angeles: Lowell House, 1998.

Blaivas, Jerry G. *Conquering Bladder and Prostate Problems: The Authoritative Guide for Men and Women.* New York: Plenum, 1998.

Chalker, Rebecca, and Kristene E. Whitmore. *Overcoming Bladder Disorders.* New York: HarperCollins, 1991.

Falcone, Ron. *Natural Medicine for Prostate Problems.* New York: Dell, 1998.

Korda, Michael. *Man to Man: Surviving Prostate Cancer.* New York: Vintage, 1997.

Loo, Marcus H., and Marian Betancourt. *The Prostate Cancer Sourcebook: How to Take Charge and Make Informed Choices.* New York: John Wiley & Sons, 1998.

National Cancer Institute. *Taking Time: Support for People With Cancer and the People Who Care About Them.* Bethesda, MD: National Institutes of Health, 1994.

Suggested Reading

Oesterling, Joseph A., and Mark A. Moyad. *The ABCs of Prostate Cancer: The Book That Could Save Your Life.* New York: Madison, 1997.

Phillips, Robert H. *Coping With Prostate Cancer.* New York: Avery, 1994.

Rous, Stephen N. *The Prostate Book: Sound Advice on Symptoms and Treatment.* New York: W.W. Norton, 1992.

Salmans, Sandra. *Prostate: Questions You Have . . . Answers You Need.* Allentown, PA: People's Medical Society, 1996.

Walsh, Patrick C., and Janet Farrar Worthington. *The Prostate: A Guide for Men and the Women Who Love Them.* New York: Warner, 1997.

Weiss, Robert E. *Management of Prostate Disease.* Lewisville, TX: J. A. Majors, 1998.

Index

A

Acute bacterial prostatitis, 23–24, 26, 27, 28, 213
Acute urinary retention, 50–51, 213
Adjuvant treatments, 153–54, 179, 213
Adrenal glands, 181, 184
African Americans, 116, 117–18, 133, 135–36
Age
    prostate cancer and, 116–17, 118
    PSA levels and, 132, 133
    radical prostatectomy and, 160–61, 164, 165
Agency for Health Care Policy and Research (AHCPR), 12, 61, 80, 85, 89
Alcohol intake, 44
Allergy medicines, 51
Allopurinol, 31
Alpha-adrenergic blockers (antihypertensives), 31, 33, 95, 96–97, 100, 102, 103, 213
Alpha-Tocopherol, Beta Carotene Cancer Prevention Study, 124
American Board of Medical Specialties (ABMS), 10
American Board of Urology, 10
American Cancer Society (ACS), 15, 16, 113, 118, 121, 127, 144, 209
    digital rectal exam recommendations of, 130
    National Prostate Cancer Detection Project of, 138–39, 140
    PSA test recommendations of, 135–36, 137
American Health, 61
American Medical Association, 117
American Osteopathic Association (AOA), 10
American Society of Hospital Pharmacists (ASHP), 163–64
American Urological Association, 61, 121, 136, 165
    BPH symptom index of, 62–63
    PSA test recommendations of, 137

INDEX

Anabolic steroids, 44
Analgesics, 32, 213
Anatomy of the prostate, 2–4
Androgens, 41, 98, 179, 181, 183, 213
    prostate cancer and, 115
    See also Testosterone
Antiandrogen, 181, 182, 213
Antibiotics, 29–30, 32, 33, 70
    blood-prostate barrier and, 25
    injection of, 33–34
Antihistamines, 51, 52, 106
Antihypertensives (alpha-adrenergic blockers), 31, 33, 95, 96–97, 100, 102, 103, 213
Anus, 27, 214
Aromatase, 95–96, 214
Aromatase inhibitors, 95, 96
Artificial insemination, 87, 214
Artificial urinary sphincter, 84–85, 214
Aspiration, 145, 214
    ultrasonic, 93, 224
Atamestane, 96

B

Back pain, 126
Bacterial prostatitis, 6, 20, 23–25, 26, 32, 214
    acute, 23–24, 26, 27, 28, 213
    chronic, 24, 28, 29, 33, 216
    treatment for, 32–35
Bactrim, 33
Balloon urethroplasty (balloon dilatation), 88–90, 214
Benign, 214
Benign prostatic hyperplasia (BPH), 6, 12, 37–58, 214
    bacterial prostatitis and, 24
    causes of, 40–43
    diagnosing, 12, 15, 52–58
    incidence of, 39–40
    PAP levels and, 148
    progression of, 46–52, 61
    PSA levels and, 132, 134
    recurrence of, 76–77
    risk factors for, 43–45
    symptoms of, 45–46, 47–52, 53, 59, 60, 61, 62–63, 64, 126
    what it is, 38–39
Benign prostatic hyperplasia (BPH), treatment for, 58, 59–108
    delaying of, 63
    differing opinions among doctors on, 60
    getting second opinion on, 64–66
    medications, 95–104
    nonsurgical, 88–95
    reasons for, 59
    self-care, 104–8
    surgery. *See* Prostatectomy, partial
    watchful waiting, 60–64
Beta carotene, 122, 214
Bicalutamide (carodex), 181
Bilateral orchiectomy (testicle removal), 159–60, 179, 181, 182, 183, 215
Biofeedback, 83, 186, 215
Biological response modifiers (BRM), 185
Biological therapies, 185–86
Biopsy, 18, 139, 144–46, 147, 148, 215
    aspiration-type, 145
    of lymph nodes, 150
    PSA levels and, 131

Birth weight, 119
Bladder, 2, 23, 24, 60, 144, 215
    benign prostatic hyperplasia and, 46–50, 52, 53–54, 55, 58
    compensated, 47, 216
    decompensated, 49, 216
Bladder catheterization, 55, 215
Blood, in urine, 7, 46, 126, 218
Blood pressure, 96–97, 102, 184
Blood-prostate barrier, 25, 215
Blood tests, 17, 50, 56, 147–48
    prostate-specific antigen. *See* Prostate-specific antigen test
    prostatic acid phosphatase (PAP), 56, 147–48, 220
Board certification, 9–10
Bone metastases, 126, 144, 146, 147, 149, 183, 201, 202, 203
Bone scan, 146, 149, 215
BPH. *See* Benign prostatic hyperplasia
Brachytherapy (interstitial radiation therapy), 174–78, 215
Brain, metastasis to, 201, 202
Breast enlargement, 98–99, 104
BRM (biological response modifiers), 185
Bruskewitz, Reginald, 98
Bush, Irving M., 106

C

Ca—A Cancer Journal for Clinicians, 127, 193
Cancer, 113
    prostate. *See* Prostate cancer
Candida, 25
Capromab pendetide (ProstaScint), 150–51
Cardura (doxazosin), 96, 103
Carodex (bicalutamide), 181
Carotenoid, 122, 215
Carter, H. Ballentine, 117, 136
Castration, 40–41, 182
    See also Hormonal therapy
Catalona, William, 132
Catheters, catheterization, 14, 55, 86, 215
    Foley, 55–56, 69, 218
CAT (computerized tomography) scan, 148, 216
Causes of prostate disease
    of benign prostatic hyperplasia, 40–43
    of prostate cancer, 115–16
    See also Risk factors
CaverMap, 166
Cellules, 48, 216
Chalker, Rebecca, 84
Chemotherapy, 185
Chlamydia, 25, 216
Chronic bacterial prostatitis, 24, 28, 29, 33, 216
Clinical trials, 195–96, 203
Coitus interruptus, 22, 216
Cold medicines, 51, 106
Colon bacilli, 24, 216
Compensated bladder, 47, 216
Complications
    from partial prostatectomy, 80–88
    from radical prostatectomy, 161–70
Computerized tomography (CT; CAT) scan, 148, 216
Concato, John, 79
Congestive prostatitis, 20–22, 221

INDEX

Creatinine, 50, 216
Cryosurgery, 216
    for benign prostatic hyperplasia, 94
    for prostate cancer, 172–73
CT (computerized tomography) scan, 148, 216
Curative therapies, 153, 216
Cystoscopy, 16–17, 18, 29, 57–58, 89, 216

D

Death rates, from prostatectomies, 77–80
Decompensated bladder, 49, 216
Decongestants, 51, 52, 106
Depression, 209–10
DHT (dihydrotestosterone), 41–42, 95, 97, 98, 100, 125–26, 217
Diabetes, 52
Diagnosing prostate disease
    benign prostatic hyperplasia, 12, 15, 52–58
    prostate cancer, 127–42
    prostatitis, 28–29
    tests in. *See* Tests
Diet
    benign prostatic hyperplasia and, 44
    prostate cancer and, 115–16, 117–19, 122–23, 188–89
Differentiation therapy, 186
Digital rectal exam (DRE), 15–16, 18, 28, 54, 127–29, 130, 136, 146, 147, 217
    combined with other tests, 140–42
    PAP levels and, 148

PSA levels and, 131–32
    recommendations for, 130
Dihydrotestosterone (DHT), 41–42, 95, 97, 98, 100, 125–26, 217
Diverticula, 48, 217
Doctor. *See* Physician
Doxazosin (Cardura), 96, 103
Dribbling (intermittency), 49, 218
Drinking, 44
Drugs. *See* Medications
Dry orgasm (retrograde ejaculation), 85–87, 221

E

Ejaculation
    painful, 126
    PSA levels and, 131
    retrograde (dry orgasm), 85–87, 221
Emotions, cancer and, 203–10
Endothelin-1 agonists, 186
Environmental factors, in prostate cancer, 124–25
Epididymis, 4, 217
Epididymitis, 88, 217
Epstein, Barry E., 167
Erection problems. *See* Impotence
Estrogen, 40, 42, 95–96, 98, 115, 217
Estrogen therapy, 104, 180, 182
Eulexin (flutamide), 181
Excretory urogram, 56–57, 217
Exercise, 125
External-beam radiotherapy, 173–74, 176–78, 217

F

Fat, dietary, 115–16, 118–19
Fertility and sterility, 5, 32, 85–87, 170

Finasteride (Proscar), 97–102, 103, 105, 125–26, 181
Fistula, 164, 217
5-alpha-reductase, 41, 99, 217
5-alpha-reductase inhibitors, 95, 97, 103
    Proscar (finasteride), 97–102, 103, 105, 125–26, 181
Flomax (tamsulosin HCl), 102, 103
Flutamide (Eulexin), 182
Foley catheter, 55–56, 69, 218
Food and Drug Administration (FDA), 91, 92, 93, 96, 98, 133, 166, 181
Foods. *See* Diet
Functions of the prostate, 4–5

G
Gene, prostate cancer, 141
Giovannucci, Edward, 122
Gland, 2, 218
Glossary, 213–25
Gonorrhea, 25, 26–27, 218
Goserelin (Zoladex), 180
Greenberger, Monroe E., 21, 22, 30
Growth factors, 42, 218
    insulin-like growth factor-1, 138
Guide to Clinical Preventive Services, 16
Gynecomastia, 98–99

H
Harvard Alumni Health Study, 125
Heart attacks, 79
Heat therapy (hyperthermia; thermotherapy), 90–92, 193, 223
Hematuria (blood in the urine), 7, 46, 126, 218

Herbicides, 124
Hesitancy, 48, 218
Homeopathy, 107
Hormonal therapy, 103–4, 153, 171, 172, 179–83, 189, 218
    candidates for, 183
    costs of, 182
    luteinizing hormone-releasing hormone analog, 180–81, 182, 219
    side effects of, 181–82
    testicle removal (orchiectomy), 159–60, 179, 181, 182, 183, 215
Hospital safety, 162–64
Human papillomavirus (HPV), 119
Hyperplasia, 37
Hyperthermia (thermotherapy; heat therapy), 90–92, 193, 223
Hytrin (terazosin), 96–97, 100–102, 103

I
Iatrogenesis, 162–63
IGF-1 (insulin-like growth factor-1), 138
Imaging, 18
Immune system, 186, 187, 208
Immunotherapy, 185, 186
Implants (interstitial radiation therapy), 174–78, 215
Impotence, 5, 27, 75, 80, 81, 82, 98, 104, 218
    after cryosurgery, 173
    after hormonal therapy, 182
    after prostatectomy, 164–67
    after radiation therapy, 174, 176
    treatments for, 168–70

Incontinence, 53, 80–85, 166, 170, 218
  products for dealing with, 86–87
  stress, 81, 82, 83, 170, 222
  treating, 82–85
Infertility, 5, 32, 85–87, 170
Informational groups, 211–12
Insulin-like growth factor-1 (IGF-1), 138
Interferons, 185–86
Intermittency, 49, 218
Interstitial radiation therapy (brachytherapy), 174–78, 215
Intravenous pyelogram (IVP; intravenous urogram; IVU), 56–57, 217

J
Journal of the American Medical Association, 78, 134, 156, 190
Journal of the National Cancer Institute, 120, 122
Journal of Urology, 31, 61, 64, 170

K
Kegel exercises, 82–83
Kidneys, 50, 57, 60
Kirkemo, Aaron, 61
Kramer, Barry, 135

L
Lancet, 128
Laparoscopy, 150, 219
Lasers, 94–95
Lee, Fred, 139, 146
Leuprolide (Lupton), 180

Lifestyle factors, in prostate cancer, 125
Luteinizing hormone-releasing hormone (LHRH) analog, 180–81, 182, 219
Lu-Yao, Grace, 164
Lymph nodes, 143, 144, 148, 149, 150, 183, 219
  radiation therapy and, 177
  radical prostatectomy and, 158, 159
Lymphadenectomy, 150, 219
Lymphangiogram, 150, 219

M
Macrobiotic diet, 188–89
Magnetic resonance imaging (MRI), 149, 219
Man to Man, 209
Manual rectal exam. *See* Digital rectal exam
Mayo Clinic, 147, 159
McGuire, Edward, 64
Medications
  antihypertensives (alpha-adrenergic blockers), 31, 33, 95, 96–97, 100, 102, 103, 213
  aromatase inhibitors, 95, 96
  for benign prostatic hyperplasia, 95–104
  errors in administering, 163–64
  5-alpha-reductase inhibitors, 95, 97–102, 103
  in hormonal therapy, 103–4
  Proscar (finasteride), 97–102, 103, 105, 125–26, 181
  for prostate cancer, 184–85

Metastases, 110, 142, 143, 144, 167, 192–93, 201–3, 219
    bone, 126, 144, 146, 147, 149, 183, 201, 202, 203
Minipress (prazosin), 31, 96
Mortality rates, from prostatectomies, 77–80
MRI (magnetic resonance imaging), 149, 219
Mutual-aid groups, 207–9, 211–12

N

Nafarelin acetate, 104, 219
National Cancer Institute (NCI), 99, 114, 116, 117, 119, 126, 140, 160, 171, 184, 194
    clinical trial recommendations of, 195–96
    Prostate Intervention Versus Observation Trial of, 154
    PSA test recommendations of, 137
    rectal exam recommendations of, 130
National Center for Health Statistics, 38
National Institutes of Health, 121
Necrosis, 91, 219
Nerve-sparing prostatectomy, 165–67, 170, 177
New England Journal of Medicine, 75, 78–79, 98, 124
Nilutamide (Nilandron), 181
Nocturia, 47, 219
Nonbacterial prostatitis, 20–23, 26, 27, 28
    treatment for, 29–32

Nonspecific urethritis (NSU), 25–26, 219
Nosocomial infection, 162–63

O

Obstructive uropathy, 64
Oesterling, Joseph, 147, 190
Official ABMS Directory of Board-Certified Medical Specialists, 66
Onik, Gary, 173
Orchiectomy (testicle removal), 159–60, 179, 181, 182, 183, 215
Orgasm, 85
    dry (retrograde ejaculation), 85–87, 221
Overcoming Bladder Disorders (Chalker and Whitmore), 84–85

P–Q

Pain management, 32, 202–3
Palliative treatments, 153, 220
PAP (prostatic acid phosphatase) test, 56, 147–48, 220
Perineal prostatectomy, 68, 71, 75, 157–58
Perineum, 27, 220
Physician
    avoidance of, 112–13
    finding, 8–12, 66
    first meeting with, 13–14
    getting second opinion from, 64–66
    hospital safety and, 162–64
    questions to ask, about cancer treatment, 155–56

Index

Physicians' Health Study, 138
Placebos, 105
Practitioner. *See* Physician
Prazosin (Minipress), 31, 96
Private Battle, A (Ryan), 110, 188
Proscar (finasteride), 97–102, 103, 105, 125–26, 181
Proscar Safety Plus Efficacy Canadian Two-Year (PROSPECT) study, 105
ProstaScint (capromab pendetide), 150–51
Prostate, 1–18, 220
    anatomy of, 2–4
    enlarged, 1, 17, 28. *See also* Benign prostatic hyperplasia
    functions of, 4–5
    growth of, 38
    lobes (zones) of, 3
    problems with. *See* Prostate disease
Prostate Book, The (Rous), 21, 40, 77, 146, 161
Prostate cancer, 1, 6–7, 27, 109–51, 220
    age and, 116–17, 118
    benign prostatic hyperplasia and, 44–45
    causes of, 115–16
    cystoscope and, 17
    determining spread of, 142–51
    diagnosing, 127–42
    diet and, 115–16, 117–19, 122–23, 188–89
    emotional impact of, 203–10
    family history of, 117, 136, 141
    gene for, 141
    growing public image of, 110–11
    incidence of, 113–15
    metastasis of, 110, 142, 143, 144, 167, 192–93, 201–3
    open prostatectomy and, 73
    preventing and slowing progress of, 121–26
    Proscar and, 99
    rectal exams and, 15, 16, 127–29, 130
    residual, 178
    risk factors for, 116–21
    stages of, 142–51, 222
    support groups for, 207–9, 211–12
    survival rates for, 144
    symptoms of, 7–8, 126–27, 146
    vasectomy and, 120–21
    what it is, 110–13
Prostate cancer, treatment for, 144, 153–210
    adjuvant, 153–54, 179, 213
    alternative, 186–89
    biological, 185–86
    choosing according to stage, 194–200
    clinical trials of, 195–96, 203
    cryosurgery, 172–73, 216
    curative, 153, 216
    drug therapy, 184–85
    emotional effects of, 203–10
    follow-up, 200–201
    hormonal therapy. *See* Hormonal therapy
    macrobiotic diet, 188–89
    nontreatment, 154
    palliative, 153, 220

questions to ask doctor about, 155–56
radiation. *See* Radiation therapy
radical prostatectomy, 150, 153, 154, 157–72, 177–78, 190. *See also* Prostatectomy, radical
recurrence of cancer following, 201–3
vaccines, 186, 187–88
watchful waiting, 154, 189–93, 194
Prostate disease, 1–2, 6–7
benign. *See* Benign prostatic hyperplasia; Prostatitis
diagnosing. *See* Diagnosing prostate disease
physician for treating. *See* Physician
symptoms of. *See* Symptoms of prostate disease
See also Benign prostatic hyperplasia; Prostate cancer; Prostatitis
Prostate Intervention Versus Observation Trial, 154
Prostate-selective alpha$_{1A}$-adrenoreceptor agonist, 102, 103
Prostate-specific antigen (PSA), 129, 138, 220
Prostate-specific antigen (PSA) test, 17, 18, 56, 99, 114–15, 129–37, 146, 147, 171, 179, 200–201
age and, 132, 133
combined with other tests, 140–42
free-state, 133–34, 146

need and optimal intervals for, 134–37
problems with, 131–35
Prostatectomy, partial (BPH surgery), 45, 60, 61, 63–64, 65, 66, 67–88, 114
closed, 67–68, 71–73, 77. *See also* Transurethral incision of the prostate; Transurethral resection of the prostate
complications from, 80–88
mortality rates from, 77–80
open, 67, 68–71, 73–75, 77–80
perineal, 68, 71, 75
postponing of, 63
prostate cancer and, 121
recovery times for, 73–74
retropubic, 68, 70–71, 75
second, 75, 76–77
suprapubic, 68, 70, 75
transurethral. *See* Transurethral incision of the prostate; Transurethral resection of the prostate
weighing options in, 71–88
Prostatectomy, radical, 221
age and, 160–61, 164, 165
candidates for, 158–61
impotence from, 164–67
nerve-sparing, 165–67, 170, 177
perineal, 157–58
for prostate cancer, 150, 153, 154, 157–72, 177–78, 190
for prostatitis, 34
recovery from, 158
retreatment following, 171–72

237

Prostatectomy, radical (*cont.*)
  retropubic, 157–58
  risks and complications of, 161–70
Prostatic acid phosphatase (PAP) test, 56, 147–48, 220
Prostatic capsule, 3
Prostatic fluid, 20–22
Prostatic urethra. *See* Urethra, prostatic
Prostatism, silent, 51–52, 222
Prostatitis, 6, 19–36, 220
  acute bacterial, 23–24, 26, 27, 28, 213
  bacterial, 6, 20, 23–25, 26, 32, 214
  chronic bacterial, 24, 28, 29, 33, 216
  congestive, 20–22, 221
  diagnosing, 28–29
  nonbacterial, 20–23, 26, 27, 28, 29–32
  PAP levels and, 148
  PSA levels and, 131
  symptoms of, 26–27
  treatment for, 29–36
  what it is, 20–26
Prostatodynia, 20, 23, 27, 31, 220
Prostatostasis (congestive prostatitis), 20–22, 221
Prostatron, 91–92
Prosthesis, 221
  artificial urinary sphincter, 84–85, 214
  for impotence, 169–70
  after testicle removal, 179
Proton therapy, 174
PSA test. *See* Prostate-specific antigen test

R

Radiation oncologist, 173
Radiation therapy (radiotherapy), 153, 171–72, 173–79, 190, 202, 203, 221
  external-beam, 173–74, 176–78, 217
  interstitial, 174–78, 215
  LHRH analogs used with, 180
  surgery vs., 177
Radical prostatectomy. *See* Prostatectomy, radical
Radiologist, 173
Radiopharmaceuticals, 202, 221
Radio-wave therapy (transurethral needle ablation; TUNA), 92–93
Reagan, Ronald, 39, 76
Recalled by Life (Sattilaro), 189
Rectal exam. *See* Digital rectal exam
Rectum, 2, 221
Reflux, 50, 221
Renal scan, 57, 221
Resectoscope, 67–68, 87, 221
Retrograde ejaculation (dry orgasm), 85–87, 221
Retropubic, 221
  prostatectomy, 68, 70–71, 75, 157–58
Risk factors
  for benign prostatic hyperplasia, 43–45
  for prostate cancer, 116–21
  See also Causes of prostate disease
Roos, Noralou, 75, 76, 77, 78, 79
Rous, Stephen N., 21, 30, 40, 77, 146, 161
Ryan, Cornelius, 110, 188

S

Safety in the hospital, 162–64
Sattilaro, Anthony J., 188, 189
Saw palmetto, 107
Science, 138
Scrotum, 4, 221
Second opinions, 64–66
Segmented urine culture, 28–29, 222
Selenium, 123
Self-injection treatment for impotence, 168, 169
Semen, 4, 5, 85
    congestive prostatitis and, 20–22
Seminal vesicles, 4–5, 222
Septra, 33
Sexually transmitted diseases, 119, 122, 125
    gonorrhea, 25, 26–27, 218
    human papillomavirus (HPV), 119
Sharlip, Ira, 23
Sildenafil (Viagra), 168
Silent prostatism, 51–52, 222
Skull, metastasis to, 201, 202
Sonogram, 138, 139, 222
    See also Ultrasound
Specialists, 8–10
Spermatozoa, 4–5, 32, 85, 170, 222
Spinal cord compression, 201, 202
Staging, 142–44, 222
    tests for, 144–51
Stent, 93, 222
Sterility and fertility, 5, 32, 85–87, 170
Steroids, 44
Stress incontinence, 81, 82, 83, 170, 222
Stricture, 222
    urethral, 52, 87–88
Stroma, 43, 222
Sulfa, 33
Sunlight, 123–24
Support groups, 207–9, 211–12
Suprapubic, 222
    prostatectomy, 68, 70, 75
Suramin, 184–85
Surgery
    for benign prostatic hyperplasia. *See* Prostatectomy, partial
    hospital safety and, 162–64
    partial prostatectomy. *See* Prostatectomy, partial
    for prostate cancer, 150, 153, 154, 157–72, 177. *See also* Prostatectomy, radical
    for prostatitis, 34
    radical prostatectomy. *See* Prostatectomy, radical
    second opinions on, 65
    testicle removal (orchiectomy), 159–60, 179, 181, 182, 183, 215
    weighing options in, 71–88
Sympathomimetic, 51, 222
Symptoms of prostate disease, 7–8
    of benign prostatic hyperplasia, 45–46, 47–52, 53, 59, 60, 61, 62–63, 64, 126
    of prostate cancer, 7–8, 126–27, 146
    of prostatitis, 26–27
    See also Urinary problems
Systemic, 223
    infection, 28

Index

T
Tamsulosin HCl (Flomax), 102, 103
Terazosin (Hytrin), 96–97, 100–102, 103
Testicles, 4, 223
    removal of (orchiectomy), 159–60, 179, 181, 182, 183, 215
Testosterone, 41, 42, 95–96, 97, 98, 223
    dihydrotestosterone, 41–42, 95, 97, 98, 100, 125–26, 217
    hormonal therapy and, 103–4, 180–81
    prostate cancer and, 115–16, 119, 125
Tests, 12–18
    blood tests, 17, 50, 56, 147–48. *See also* Prostate-specific antigen test
    combining, 140–42
    cystoscopy, 16–17, 18, 29, 57–58, 89, 216
    PSA test. *See* Prostate-specific antigen test
    rectal exam. *See* Digital rectal exam
    renal scan, 57, 221
    second opinions on, 66
    for staging prostate cancer, 144–51
    transrectal ultrasonography, 136, 137–39, 140–42, 145, 148, 223
    ultrasound, 57, 136, 137–39, 145, 146, 148
    urinalysis, 14, 18, 28, 32, 54, 224
    urine culture, 28–29, 32, 54, 225
    urodynamic studies, 53, 54–55, 225
Thermotherapy (hyperthermia; heat therapy), 90–92, 193, 223
Tomatoes, 122
Trabeculation, 48, 58, 223
Transrectal microwave hyperthermia, 90–91, 92, 193, 223
Transrectal ultrasound (TRUS), 136, 137–39, 145, 148, 223
    combined with other tests, 140–42
Transurethral incision of the prostate (TUIP), 67, 68, 71–73, 223
    complications from, 80, 85, 87, 88
    cost of, 72–73
    deciding between TURP and, 71–73
    what to expect after, 69–70
Transurethral microwave thermotherapy (TUMT), 90, 91–92, 93, 223
Transurethral needle ablation (TUNA), 92–93
Transurethral resection of the prostate (TURP), 64, 67–68, 71, 72–75, 224
    complications from, 80, 81, 85, 87–88
    cost of, 72–73
    deciding between TUIP and, 71–73
    mortality rate from, 77–80
    prostate cancer and, 192–93
    what to expect after, 69–70

Transurethral ultrasound-guided
  laser-induced prostatectomy
  (TULIP), 94–95, 224
Treatments
  for benign prostatic hyperplasia.
    See Benign prostatic
    hyperplasia, treatment for
  for prostate cancer. *See* Prostate
    cancer, treatment for
  for prostatitis, 29–36
Trimethoprim, 33
TRUS (transrectal ultrasound), 136,
  137–39, 145, 148, 223
  combined with other tests,
    140–42
TUIP. *See* Transurethral incision of
  the prostate
TULIP (transurethral
  ultrasound-guided laser-induced
  prostatectomy), 94–95, 224
Tumor, Nodes, Metastases (TNM)
  System, 143
TUMT (transurethral microwave
  thermotherapy), 90, 91–92,
  93, 223
TUNA (transurethral needle
  ablation), 92–93
TURP. *See* Transurethral resection of
  the prostate

U

Ultrasonic aspiration, 93, 224
Ultrasound, 57, 146, 224
  transrectal, 136, 137–39,
    140–42, 145, 148, 223
  transurethral ultrasound-guided
    laser-induced prostatectomy,
    94–95

Urea nitrogen, 50, 224
Uremic poisoning (uremia), 50, 224
Ureters, 54, 224
Urethra, 2, 39, 224
  gonorrhea and, 26–27
Urethra, prostatic, 2, 5, 81, 220
  balloon dilatation of,
    88–90, 214
  benign prostatic hyperplasia
    and, 39, 43, 46, 50, 52, 54,
    57, 64
  prostatectomy and, 67
  urethritis and, 25–26, 29
Urethral sphincter, 2–3, 23, 81, 224
Urethral stricture, 52, 87–88
Urethritis, 25–26, 29, 219
Urinalysis, 14, 18, 28, 32, 54, 224
Urinary problems, 7, 52
  alleviating, 104–6, 107
  in benign prostatic hyperplasia,
    37–38, 45–53, 54–56,
    57–58, 59, 60, 62–63, 64
  blood in the urine, 7, 46,
    126, 218
  hesitancy, 48, 218
  incontinence. *See* Incontinence
  intermittency, 49, 218
  medications as cause of, 51,
    52, 106
  nocturia, 47, 219
  in prostate cancer, 126, 146
  in prostatitis, 27
Urinary retention, 14, 225
  acute, 50–51, 213
Urinary sphincter, artificial,
  84–85, 214
Urine culture, 32, 54, 225
  segmented, 28–29, 222

Urodynamic studies, 53, 54–55, 225
Uroflometer, 54, 225
Urologist, 8, 11, 12, 225
Urology, 96, 101, 129
UroLume Endoprosthesis, 93
Uropathy, obstructive, 64
U.S. Preventive Services Task Force, 130, 136, 137
US TOO, 209

V

Vaccines, prostate cancer, 186, 187–88
Vacuum devices, 168, 169
Vas deferens, 4, 170, 225
Vasectomy, 120–21, 225
Viagra (sildenafil), 168
Visualization, 186
Vitamin D, 123, 124
Vitamin E, 124

W

Walsh, Patrick, 165, 170
Wasson, John H., 64

Watchful waiting
   for benign prostatic hyperplasia, 60–64
   for prostate cancer, 154, 189–93, 194
Weight, 125
Wennberg, John, 60, 76, 77
What Every Man Should Know About His Prostate (Greenberger), 21
Whitmore, Kristene E., 84
Whitmore, Willet F., Jr., 154, 156

X

X-rays, 17, 56, 146
   computerized tomography scan, 148, 216
   excretory urogram, 56–57, 217

Y

Yeast infection, 25

Z

Zinc, 34–35, 106
Zoladex (goserelin), 180